Hot Health Care Careers

College & Caree
Chicago, Illin

Editorial Staff

Andrew Morkes, Publisher/Managing Editor/Writer
Amy McKenna, Publisher/Editor
Felicitas Cortez, Writer/Editor
Nora Walsh, Writer/Editor
Jon Bieniek, Proofreader
Kevin Meyers Design, Cover Design

Library of Congress Cataloging-in-Publication Data
Morkes, Andrew.
  Hot health care careers : more than 25 cutting-edge jobs with the fastest growth
and most new positions / by Andrew Morkes and Amy McKenna.
      p. cm.
  Includes bibliographical references and index.
  Summary: "Provides an overview of more than 25 health care careers that have
been identified by the U.S. Department of Labor as offering the fastest employment growth and the most new jobs through 2018. Each article provides an
overview of job duties, educational requirements, interviews with workers in the
field, and more"--Provided by publisher.
  ISBN 978-0-9745251-5-0
  1. Medical personnel--Vocational guidance. I. McKenna, Amy, 1969- II. Title.
  R690.M595 2011
  610.69023--dc22

                                    2010032797

Published and distributed by
College & Career Press, LLC
PO Box 300484
Chicago, IL 60630
773/282-4671 (phone/fax)
amorkes@chicagopd.com
www.collegeandcareerpress.com

Printed in the United States of America

01-11

TABLE OF CONTENTS

INTRODUCTION

Health care jobs are a popular career option for students who enjoy help-ing others and learning about the latest cutting-edge technology and treatment methods! The health care industry is one of the few industries that is actually growing during these tough economic times. In fact, the U.S. Department of Labor (USDL) predicts that employment in the health care industry will grow by 22 percent—double the average employment growth for all industries. It also reports that 12 of the top 20 fastest-grow-ing careers through 2018 are in the health care industry. No other indus-try will add more jobs than the health care field from 2008-18. In fact, the USDL predicts that the growing elderly population, expansion of health insurance by the federal government, and technological breakthroughs will help generate 3.2 million new jobs between 2008 and 2018. Nine of the top 20 careers that will add the most new positions through 2018 are in the health care industry, according to the USDL. These predictions adds up to an excellent outlook for many health care careers.

The editors of *Hot Health Care Careers* have chosen 26 careers that will grow most quickly and add the most new jobs through 2018. These careers offer exciting opportunities for people with a variety of skill sets and educational backgrounds—from a high school diploma and on-the-job training, to a bachelor's or master's degree, to a medical degree, den-tal degree, or doctorate. The following paragraphs provide more informa-tion on the sections in each career article and other features in the book.

The **Fast Facts** sidebar appears at the beginning of each article. It pro-vides a summary of recommended high school classes and personal skills; the minimum educational requirements to enter the field; the typical salary range; employment outlook; and acronyms and identification numbers for the following government classification indexes: the Occupational Information Network (O*NET)-Standard Occupational Classification System (SOC) index; the Guide for Occupational Exploration (GOE); the Dictionary of Occupational Titles (DOT); and the National Occupational Classification (NOC) Index. The O*NET-SOC, GOE, and DOT indexes have been created by the U.S. government; the NOC index is Canada's career classification system. Readers can use the identification numbers listed in this section to obtain further information about a career. Print edi-tions of the GOE (*Guide for Occupational Exploration*. Indianapolis, Ind.: JIST Works, 2001) and DOT (*Dictionary of Occupational Titles*. Indianapolis, Ind.: JIST Works, 1991) are available at libraries. Electronic versions of the DOT (www.oalj.dol.gov/libdot.htm), NOC (www5.hrsdc.gc.ca/NOC), and O*NET-SOC (http://online.onetcenter.org) are available on the Internet. When no O*NET-SOC, GOE, DOT, or NOC numbers are listed, this means that the U.S. Department of Labor or Human Resources and Skills Development Canada have not created a numerical designation for this career. In this instance, you will see the acronym "N/A," or not available.

The **Overview** section provides a capsule summary of work duties, educational requirements, the number of people employed in the field, and employment outlook.

The Job provides a detailed overview of primary and secondary job duties and typical work settings.

The **Requirements** section features four subsections: **High School** (which lists recommended high school classes), **Postsecondary Training** (which lists required post-high school training requirements to prepare for the field), **Certification and Licensing** (which details voluntary certification and mandatory licensing requirements, when applicable), and **Other Requirements** (which lists key personal and professional skills for success in the field).

Exploring provides suggestions to young people about how they can explore the field while in school. Examples include books and magazines, websites, information interviews, membership in clubs and other organizations, hands-on activities, competitions, and summer and after-school programs.

Employers lists the number of people employed in the occupation in the United States and details typical work settings.

Getting a Job provides advice on how to land a job through employment and association websites, career service offices, networking, career fairs, and other methods.

The **Advancement** section provides an overview of typical ways to move up at one's employer or via other means (such as opening a consulting firm or entering academia).

Earnings provides information on starting, median, and top salaries for workers. Information on salaries in particular industries is also provided for many careers.

The **Employment Outlook** section provides an overview of the outlook for the career through 2018. It lists the factors that are causing employment to grow and details career areas in which there will be especially strong growth. Outlook information is obtained from the U.S. Department of Labor and is augmented by information gathered from professional trade associations. Job growth terms follow those used in the *Occupational Outlook Handbook* (http://stats.bls.gov/search/ooh.htm). Growth described as "much faster than the average" means that employment will increase by 20 percent or more from 2008 to 2018. Growth described as "faster than the average" means an increase of 14 to 19 percent. Growth described as "about as fast as the average" means an increase of 7 to 13 percent.

Each article ends with **For More Information.** This section provides contact information for professional associations that provide details on educational programs, career paths, scholarships, publications, youth programs, and other resources.

Additionally, most articles in *Hot Health Care Careers* feature one or more interviews with professionals and educators, who provide useful advice on what it takes to land a job and be successful. Other features include informative sidebars, photographs, and a career title and association index.

We hope that *Hot Health Care Careers* provides you with some great ideas for possible career paths. But this book is just the beginning. Contact the professional associations listed at the end of each article to obtain more information; perhaps they can even help arrange an information interview with a worker in a field that interests you. Follow the suggestions in the Exploring section of each article to get hands-on experience. That way, you will be able to try out each field before making the big decision of choosing a career. Learning about health care careers can be fun, and we hope this book is useful to you as you begin your search. All the best to you during your career exploration!

ADVANCED PRACTICE NURSES

OVERVIEW

Advanced practice nurses (APNs) are registered nurses who provide specialized health care, promote health, prevent and treat disease and injuries, and help patients cope with illness. APNs have earned master's degrees and certifications to become either a *certified nurse-midwife,* a *clinical nurse specialist,* a *certified registered nurse anesthetist,* or a *nurse practitioner.* There are more than 259,500 advanced practice nurses employed in the United States. Employment for APNs is expected to be excellent through 2018.

THE JOB

What makes nurses unique from other health care professionals? Many agree it is the job of the nurse to treat the individual—not just the presenting health problem. In addition, nurses are often tasked with caring not only for the patient, but for his or her loved ones and family, keeping them comfortable and "in the know" about a health crisis of a loved one. Finally, nurses are stewards in their community, keeping the public informed on ways to get and stay healthy. Advanced practice nursing is an umbrella term given to registered nurses who have completed a master's degree and passed additional clinical practice requirements specific to their chosen career path. Advanced practice nursing specialties are detailed in the following paragraphs:

Certified nurse-midwives (CNMs) provide gynecological wellness checks and consultations on conception and pregnancy, and they assist in childbirth. Approximately 7.4 percent of U.S. births are attended by certified nurse-midwives. CNMs work in hospitals and birthing centers, and they conduct home visits for women who want to deliver their babies at home. The common misconception is that all these professionals do is deliver babies. In fact, they spend only about 10 percent of their workday assist-

---

FAST FACTS

High School Subjects
Biology
Chemistry
Mathematics

Personal Skills
Active listening
Communication
Critical thinking
Judgment and decision making

Minimum Education Level
Master's degree

Salary Range
$71,000 to $100,000 to $174,000+

Employment Outlook
Much faster than the average

O*NET-SOC
29-1111.00

GOE
14.02.01

DOT
075

NOC
3152, 3232

ing in childbirth. The majority of their work involves providing routine annual exams and giving primary, preventive care to women of all ages.

Clinical nurse specialists (CNSs) specialize in a wide range of physical and mental health areas. Their area of clinical expertise may be in a setting such as emergency room nursing, a type of health problem such as stress or wounds, a population such as pediatrics or the elderly, or a type of care such as rehabilitation. In addition to direct care, they may serve as consultants, researchers, educators, and medical administrators. CNSs work in clinics, offices, community centers, hospitals, and other medical facilities.

Nurse anesthesia is the oldest advanced nursing specialty. *Certified registered nurse anesthetists (CRNAs)* administer anesthesia to patients undergoing surgery or other medical treatments. They also provide pain management and emergency services. CRNAs administer approximately 30 million anesthetics to patients annually in the United States. Men make up 44 percent of nurse anesthetists, according to the American Association of Nurse Anesthetists. Fewer than 10 percent of workers in all nursing fields are men. CRNAs work alongside surgeons, anesthesiologists, dentists, podiatrists, and other health care professionals in hospitals, in medical offices, and in other settings.

Nurse practitioners (NPs) are qualified to provide some of the direct health care services that are generally performed by physicians. They treat illnesses ranging from the common cold to diabetes. NPs have a variety of duties, including diagnosing and treating minor illnesses or injuries and prescribing medication. They also conduct physical examinations; provide immunizations; help patients manage high blood pressure, diabetes, depression, and other chronic health problems; prescribe medications; perform certain medical procedures; order and interpret lab results, x-rays, and EKGs; and educate and counsel patients and their families. Nurse practitioners can write prescriptions in all 50 states and practice independently from physicians in nearly 20 states. While many NPs focus on primary care, others—with additional training—become *pediatric, gerontological, oncology, neonatal, acute care, school, occupational health, psychiatric,* and *women's health care nurse practitioners.* NPs work in hospitals, offices of physicians, clinics, nursing homes, pharmacies with health clinics, and other medical facilities.

Work settings for advanced practice nurses vary based on their specialty, but they generally work in medical offices or hospitals. Since there is a 24-hour demand for health care, some of these professionals work nights, weekends, and holidays. Regardless of the shift, APNs find their work rewarding. They enjoy caring for patients and their families and promoting wellness education in the field and in the community.

REQUIREMENTS

High School

Take health, mathematics, biology, chemistry, physics, English, speech, business, and sociology classes in high school to prepare for a career in advanced practice nursing.

Calling Dr. Nurse!

The nursing field is adding yet another specialty—doctor of nursing practice, or DrNP. DrNPs are graduates of a two-year doctoral program (that includes a one-year residency), which advocates believe allows them to enter the medical field with the training, skill, and medical experience of a primary care physician. There were 5,165 students enrolled in DrNP programs throughout the country in 2009—an 83 percent increase from 2006, according to the American Association of Colleges of Nursing.

POSTSECONDARY TRAINING

The first step to become an APN is to complete training to become a registered nurse. Prospective RNs have the option of pursuing one of three training paths: associate's degree, diploma, and bachelor's degree. Associate's degree programs in nursing last two years and are offered by community colleges. Diploma programs in nursing typically last three years and are offered by hospitals and independent schools. Bachelor of science in nursing programs are offered by colleges and universities. They typically take four—and sometimes five—years to complete. Graduates of all three paths are known as graduate nurses and must take a licensing exam in their state to obtain the RN designation. Visit Discover Nursing (www.discovernursing.com) for a database of nursing programs.

Graduates of midwifery education programs must have a master's degree in order to be able to take the national certifying exam, which is offered by the American Midwifery Certification Board (www.amcbmidwife.org). The Accreditation Commission for Midwifery Education has accredited nearly 40 nurse-midwifery education programs in the United States. Visit www.midwife.org/map.cfm for a list of programs.

Clinical nurse specialists need at least a master's degree to work in the field. The National Association of Clinical Nurse Specialists offers a list of educational programs at its website, www.nacns.org.

Nurse anesthetists must have at least a master's degree to practice. The Council of Accreditation of Nurse Anesthesia Educational Programs has accredited more than 100 programs. Visit the American Association of Nurse Anesthetists' website, www.aana.com, for a list of programs.

You will need a master's degree to work as a nurse practitioner. Visit the website (www.aanp.org) of the American Academy of Nurse Practitioners for a database of education programs.

Doctorate degrees (such as a Doctor of Nursing Practice) are typically required for those who want to work in top levels of administration, in research, or in education. These degrees normally take four to five years to complete.

CERTIFICATION AND LICENSING

Voluntary certification is available for all four advanced practice nursing specialties. The American Midwifery Certification Board offers certification to midwives. Clinical nurse specialists can become certified by the American Nurses Credentialing Center (ANCC), the American Association of Critical

Care Nurses Certification Corporation, the Oncology Nursing Certification Corporation, and the Orthopaedic Nurses Certification Board. Nurse anesthetists can become certified by the Council on Certification of Nurse Anesthetists and the American Society of PeriAnesthesia Nurses. Nurse practitioners can obtain certification from such organizations as the American Academy of Nurse Practitioners, the ANCC, the American Nurses Association, the Oncology Nursing Certification Corporation, and the Pediatric Nursing Certification Board. Contact these organizations for more information.

Nurses must be licensed to practice nursing in all states and the District of Columbia. Licensure requirements vary by state, but they typically include graduating from an approved nursing school and passing a national examination. Visit the National Council of State Boards of Nursing's website, www.ncsbn.org, for details on licensing requirements by state.

OTHER REQUIREMENTS

Successful APNs are detail oriented, caring, sympathetic, responsible, and emotionally stable. They need excellent communication skills in order to interact well with patients and coworkers. They have good judgment, are able to remain calm and decisive under pressure, have good leadership abilities, and are willing to continue to learn and upgrade their skills throughout their careers.

Did You Know?

✔ Certified nurse midwives (CNMs) and certified midwives (CMs) attended 7.3 percent of all births in 2007.

✔ More than 82 percent of CNMs and CMs have a master's degree; 7.5 percent hold a doctoral degree.

✔ In 2008, slightly more than 53 percent of CNMs/CMs identified reproductive care as their main practice responsibility; 33.1 percent cited primary care.

Source: American College of Nurse-Midwives

EXPLORING

Read books about nursing, talk with your counselor or teacher about setting up a presentation by a nurse, take a tour of a hospital or other health care setting, or volunteer at one of these facilities. Nursing-related websites, including those of professional associations, can also be a good source of information. Here are a few suggestions: Cybernurse.com (www.cybernurse.com), Discover Nursing (www.discovernursing.com), and Nurse.com (www.nurse.com).

EMPLOYERS

There are more than 259,500 advanced practice nurses employed in the United States. Fifty-two percent of this total work as nurse practitioners, 27 percent as clinical nurse specialists, 17 percent as nurse anesthetists, and

4 percent as certified nurse-midwives. The following paragraphs provide information on work settings for the four advanced practice nursing specialties.

Certified nurse-midwives work in hospitals and birthing centers, and they conduct home visits for women who want to deliver their babies at home.

Clinical nurse specialists are employed in clinics, offices, community centers, hospitals, and other medical facilities.

Certified registered nurse anesthetists work in hospitals; outpatient surgery centers; and offices of dentists, ophthalmologists, plastic surgeons, podiatrists, and pain management specialists.

Nurse practitioners are employed in hospitals, clinics, nursing homes, mental health centers, colleges and universities, student health centers, home health agencies, hospices, offices of physicians, community health centers, rural health clinics, prisons, and industrial organizations.

Advanced practice nurses also work for government agencies, including the U.S. Department of Veterans Affairs, the U.S. Public Health Service, and the U.S. military. They also teach at colleges and universities.

GETTING A JOB

Many APNs obtain their first jobs as a result of contacts made through college internships or networking events. Others seek assistance in obtaining job leads from college career services offices, nursing registries, nurse employment agencies, state employment offices, newspaper want ads, and employment websites. Additionally, professional nursing associations (such as the National Association of Clinical Nurse Specialists and the American Academy of Nurse Practitioners) provide job listings at their websites. See For More Information for a list of organizations. Those interested in positions with the federal government should visit the U.S. Office of Personnel Management's website, www.usajobs.opm.gov.

ADVANCEMENT

The position of advanced practice nurse is not an entry-level career. Most APNs enter the field after working as registered nurses and obtaining several years of experience and advanced education and certification. APNs can eventually advance to managerial or senior-level administrative roles. These positions often require APNs to earn a doctorate degree in nursing or management. The U.S. Department of Labor reports that some APNs are hired by hospitals, pharmaceutical manufacturers, insurance companies, and managed care organizations to provide health planning and development, policy development, marketing, consulting, and quality assurance consulting. Other APNs work as teachers at colleges, universities, and teaching hospitals.

EARNINGS

Median annual salaries for registered nurses were $63,750 in 2009, according to the U.S. Department of Labor. Salaries ranged from less than $43,970 to $93,700 or more. Salaries for APNs are typically higher. Salary.com reports the following salary ranges for APNs by specialty in October 2010: certified nurse-midwives,

$76,650 to $105,604; clinical nurse specialists, $71,536 to $100,417; nurse anesthetists, $135,421 to $174,889; and nurse practitioners, $74,793 to $101,029.

APNs usually receive benefits such as health and life insurance, vacation days, sick leave, and a savings and pension plan. Self-employed workers must provide their own benefits.

EMPLOYMENT OUTLOOK

Employment for registered nurses is expected to be excellent through 2018, according to the U.S. Department of Labor (USDL). The USDL reports that these professionals "will be in high demand, particularly in medically underserved areas such as inner cities and rural areas. Relative to physicians, these RNs increasingly serve as lower-cost primary care providers." APNs with doctoral degrees and certification will have the best employment prospects.

FOR MORE INFORMATION

For information on opportunities for men in nursing, contact
**American Assembly
for Men in Nursing**
PO Box 130220
Birmingham, AL 35213-0220
www.aamn.org

For information on accredited nursing programs, contact
**American Association
of Colleges of Nursing**
One Dupont Circle, NW, Suite 530
Washington, DC 20036-1135
www.aacn.nche.edu

For certification information, contact
**American Nurses
Credentialing Center**
c/o American Nurses Association
8515 Georgia Avenue, Suite 400
Silver Spring, MD 20910-3492
www.nursecredentialing.org

For information on gerontological advanced practice nursing, contact
**Gerontological Advanced
Practice Nurses Association**
East Holly Avenue, Box 56
Pitman, NJ 08071-1735
www.gapna.org

For general information about nursing, contact
National League for Nursing
61 Broadway, 33rd Floor
New York, NY 10006-2701
800-669-1656
www.nln.org

For information on membership, contact
**National Student
Nurses' Association**
45 Main Street, Suite 606
Brooklyn, NY 11201-1099
nsna@nsna.org
www.nsna.org

For resources for aspiring and current nurses with disabilities, visit
ExceptionalNurse.com
www.exceptionalnurse.com

NURSE-MIDWIVES
For information on education, careers, and certification for certified nurse-midwives, contact the following organizations
**American College
of Nurse-Midwives**
8403 Colesville Road, Suite 1550
Silver Spring, MD 20910-6374
www.midwife.org

continued on page 7

continued from page 6

**American Midwifery
Certification Board**
849 International Drive, Suite 205
Linthicum, MD 21090-2228
www.accmidwife.org

**Midwives Alliance
of North America**
611 Pennsylvania Avenue, SE, #1700
Washington, DC 20003-4303
info@mana.org
www.mana.org

CLINICAL NURSE SPECIALISTS
For information on education and
careers, contact
**National Association
of Clinical Nurse Specialists**
100 North 20th Street, 4th Floor
Philadelphia, PA 19103-1462
www.nacns.org

NURSE ANESTHETISTS
For information on education,
careers, and certification, contact
the following organizations
**American Association
of Nurse Anesthetists**
222 South Prospect Avenue
Park Ridge, IL 60068-4037
www.aana.com

**American Society of
PeriAnesthesia Nurses**
90 Frontage Road
Cherry Hill, NJ 08034-1424
www.aspan.org

NURSE PRACTITIONERS
For more info on education and careers,
contact the following organizations
**American Academy
of Nurse Practitioners**
PO Box 12846
Austin, TX 78711-2846
www.aanp.org

**American College
of Nurse Practitioners**
1501 Wilson Boulevard, Suite 509
Arlington, VA 22209-2403
www.acnpweb.org

**National Association of Nurse
Practitioners in Women's Health**
505 C Street, NE
Washington, DC 20002-5809
www.npwh.org

**National Association
of Pediatric Nurse Practitioners**
20 Brace Road, Suite 200
Cherry Hill, NJ 08034-2634
www.napnap.org

Interview: Peggy Barksdale

Peggy Barksdale, M.S.N., RN, OCNS-C, CNS-BC is a clinical nurse specialist in orthopaedics for the Community Health Network in Indianapolis, Indiana. She discussed her career with the editors of *Hot Health Care Careers*.

Q. How long have you worked in the field? What made you want to enter this career?

A. I have worked as a nurse for 32 years and as a clinical nurse specialist for five years. My first degree was in art history, but I always loved math and science. The desire to become a nurse began around age 13, just before entering high school. I was artistic and I had an aversion to bright red blood. My counselor steered me to the arts. My husband encouraged me to try nursing. I pursued the dream in small steps. I became a licensed practical nurse, then completed being a registered nurse, and went further towards a master's degree.

Q. Can you please describe a day in your life on the job as a CNS?

A. My day is anything but typical. I am autonomous so I make my own schedule and directions for work. The clinical nurse specialist practices in three spheres, which involves the patient who is always first, then the nurses, and the system which for me that includes three hospitals. I facilitate meetings, attend conferences, and consult on patients who are difficult health wise or personality, read up on the latest in medical research, write up policies and standards of care, and find time to speak to the community and professional organizations, as well as publish articles. One responsibility that I do weekly is conduct multidisciplinary rounds at each hospital. This encompasses the attendance of the nurses, managers along with staff, pharmacists, social workers or case managers, and dietitians; even chaplains discuss each patient's hospitalization. Some of these rounds are simple and others can be moderate to very difficult in many ways. My work is 24/7. It is rare that I am called in the middle of the night or on the weekend.

Q. What are the most important qualities for CNSs?

A. The most important professional quality is expertise and knowledge regarding the clinical nurse specialist's specialty. Mine is orthopaedics. I have obtained credentials in advanced certifications in musculoskeletal conditions and as a board certified advanced practice nurse. Even the number of years in which I worked doing direct patient care helps a lot; there must be knowledge to support decisions that I make. That comes from graduate studies at the university and attending or presenting at national organizations and conferences.

Personally, the quality of leadership that builds on establishing relationships is key. Present a good first impression, maintain integrity, and be positive. For me, being optimistic is vital.

Q. What are some of the pros and cons of your job?

A. The "pros" are numerous. I love my job. I am creative in my assignments and tasks. I meet many diverse and unique people from the bedside to the boardrooms. I am a part of nursing leadership. I actively mentor others to pursue this vocation.

The "cons" means that I can be spread too thin or have to forfeit some projects for more immediate demands. My time at three campuses has its restrictions. I learn to share and at times my work can be less than perfect. Also, I am not the fastest keyboarder to [complete] paperwork needs. I sometimes mis-schedule appointments or forget when I become involved with practice situations.

Q. What advice would you give to young people who are interested in the field?

A. The advice that I would give young people who are interested in this field is to pursue your dream. I did despite a detour along the career path. Dabble in nursing's numerous specialties, such as cardiac, infants, trauma, or broken bones. Allow a passion to develop and flourish in becoming the best that you can be in that field. Learning is ongoing. What was great last month may be ancient today. Absorb challenge and be ready to change yourself or the practice of health care.

Q. What is the employment outlook for clinical nurse specialists (CNSs)?

A. The employment outlook for clinical nurse specialists is most promising. Advanced practice registered nurses are in high demand due to the experience, expertise, and their graduate-level training. These qualities contribute to promising outcomes in patient care. Less infections, injuries, and mistakes are made because the critical thinking of these experts. In today's health care reform it is about quality and successful management of diseases and chronic conditions. The supply is lower than the demand to fill positions for CNSs. Hospitals that are awarded significant recognition employ CNSs to influence safety and high-quality patient care.

Interview: Nina Ortegon

Nina Ortegon is a nurse practitioner in the Pediatric Intensive Care Unit at Advocate Hope Children's Hospital in Oak Lawn, Illinois. She discussed her career with the editors of *Hot Health Care Careers*.

Q. What made you want to enter this career?

A. I always wanted to be a nurse and after becoming a nurse, I wanted to advance in the profession and obtain my nurse practitioner (NP) certification. I wanted the opportunity to help people in the time of need and make an impact on their lives.

Q. What are the most important qualities for nurse practitioners?

A. A nurse practitioner has to have a strong nursing foundation. It is important to develop your basic nursing skills before moving on to an NP program. An NP also has to be independent and confident enough to care for patients on their own. It is also important for the NP to know when to ask for help. The NP can't be afraid to collaborate with his or her supervising doctor. The NP also has to be compassionate and have the desire to make a difference in his or her patients' lives.

My motto is to treat every patient like I would like my family treated. I also believe it is important to take my time when interacting with my patients. I want to provide the bedside manner that makes my patients know that I am there to listen and address their needs.

Q. What do you like most and least about your job?

A. I love having the opportunity to care for people in their time of need. I enjoy saving people's lives and making them feel better. I like the challenge in figuring out what is wrong with patients. At times you feel like a detective. I also enjoy treating patients' illnesses.

I dislike the fact that many hospitals are overcrowded and busy, which makes it difficult to provide the quality care that you would like to provide with every patient. You can't always spend the extra five to 10 minutes explaining something to the patient or family because you have many other patients that need to be seen. It is also hard to see people in pain or dealing with death.

Q.   What advice would you give to young people?

A.   Take science classes, and continue to work on your people skills. It is also helpful to learn a foreign language, since many of the patient populations don't speak English. After you enter college, I would recommend getting your undergraduate nursing degree. I would work as an RN for several years before starting any graduate classes. You need to find the area of nursing that you enjoy before starting with your advanced nursing education.

Q.   What is the employment outlook for nurse practitioners?

A.   There are many jobs available as an NP. You have the opportunity to work in various settings, as well. As a NP, you always have the option to work as a RN as a backup plan. Being a NP opens so many more doors for your career as a nurse.

Interview: Tara Seider

Tara Seider is a pediatric nurse at Children's Memorial Hospital in Chicago. She is currently studying to become a pediatric nurse practitioner. She discussed her career and her educational journey with the editors of *Hot Health Care Careers*.

Q.   What made you want to become a nurse? Can you tell us what prompted you to decide to transition from work as an RN to an advanced practice nurse (APN)?

A.   I have always loved the idea of helping others. Nursing seemed to be a natural fit for me.

I decided to advance my nursing career because I realized I had more to give. Being a staff/bedside nurse is wonderful and an honor, but I know with an advanced degree I can use the knowledge that I obtain to better serve my patients. I am also excited at the prospects of more responsibility and autonomy that the APN role will provide.

Q.   Can you tell us a little about your training to become an APN?

A.   I am just starting! I have three classes completed and a whole lot left. I will be taking theory classes, as well as science courses. I will also work alongside a current APN and learn hands on.

Q.   What are the most important qualities for nurses?

A.   Personal: One must have compassion, honesty, and a good sense of humor! A good nurse should be flexible and be able to relate to all types of people.

Professional: One should have integrity, good judgment, excellent communication skills, and patience.

Q.   What advice would you give to young people?

A.   Enjoy it! Be honest to your patients, be good to yourself, and take care of you. Study and ask many questions.

ATHLETIC TRAINERS

OVERVIEW

Athletic trainers, also known as *sports trainers,* help in the prevention and treatment of injuries. They treat people of all ages. Trainers work under the supervision of a physician. Their duties include the design and implementation of conditioning and strengthening programs, injury management and rehabilitation, and education and counseling, as well as administrative tasks. Many athletic trainers work with athletes—ranging from the professional to the recreational player, at all age levels. Others work with people with musculoskeletal injuries and those seeking conditioning, strength, fitness, and performance enhancement. Some trainers work in industrial settings or the performing arts. Athletic trainers must have at least a bachelor's degree in ath-

FAST FACTS

High School Subjects
Health
Physical education

Personal Skills
Critical thinking
Helping
Judgment and decision making
Organizational

Minimum Education Level
Bachelor's degree

Salary Range
$25,000 to $41,000 to $65,000+

Employment Outlook
Much faster than the average

O*NET-SOC
29-9091.00

GOE
14.08.01

DOT
153

NOC
4167

letic training or a related major to work in the field. Approximately 26,000 athletic trainers are members of the National Athletic Trainers' Association. Employment for athletic trainers is expected to be good during the next decade.

THE JOB

Athletic trainers are committed to the prevention and treatment of injuries, many of which are incurred by athletes. Their main focus is to bring the individual to an optimum fitness level to best avoid injuries and achieve overall health. When working with a new client, athletic trainers will start with an assessment, or complete physical exam, to identify any potentially dangerous abnormalities or diseases such as a heart murmur or diabetes. They may also suggest a stress test to gauge a client's cardiovascular fitness or work with weights and other exercise machines to determine a client's flexibility range. Clients may also be asked to lift a variety of weights to show their strength and endurance. Athletic trainers use a combination of scales, pincers, and computer programs to identify and analyze their client's body composition.

Once the assessment is complete, the athletic trainer designs a specific conditioning or strengthening program best suited to the client's needs. If a track-and-field athlete wants to increase his or her speed and agility, for example, the trainer could implement a series of exercises to strengthen the client's leg muscles, or use equipment such as a harness, tether, or band while the athlete is running to build endurance and strength. Athletic trainers also discuss proper nutrition and diet with their clients and may confer with a nutritionist if a special diet is needed.

Athletic trainers believe that careful preparation is key to avoiding potential injury. They inspect the facility or playing field for any potential hazards, and they check equipment for proper maintenance. For a client who is a hockey goalie, they may recommend extra protective equipment—bandage wraps, tape, or helmets and pads—to reduce the risk of injury. If needed, they suggest the use of custom devices such as special mouth guards or plastic goggles and facemasks. Athletic trainers also take the environment into consideration. When helping a football player with conditioning during the summer months, trainers may be extra diligent about their client's hydration levels or electrolyte levels during hot, humid weather, for example, and may insist on frequent water breaks and shorter workout sessions.

Unfortunately, sometimes injuries cannot be avoided—regardless of the conditioning of the individual. When an injury occurs, athletic trainers administer immediate treatment. They place ice packs to minimize a bruise, tape a sprained ankle, or clean and bandage a cut or scrape. For major injuries, the athletic trainer may need to control bleeding or regulate body temperature, or perhaps even administer CPR to restart the individual's heart and restore breathing while waiting for emergency health professionals to arrive on the scene.

Athletic trainers also help athletes regain their conditioning after an injury. Depending on the type of injury, they recommend various treatments, including massage and joint mobilization to improve flexibility and range of motion; running or rowing to improve cardiorespiratory fitness; or working with weights and balls to improve strength and balance. They may also monitor the athlete's response to medications that have been prescribed by a physician.

Athletic trainers also have administrative duties such as maintaining a client's medical records, keeping track of procedures and fitness programs, and staying up to date with the client's medications and special diets. Many athletic trainers are responsible for purchasing supplies and new fitness equipment for their facilities.

Athletic trainers are in constant communication with team coaches and physicians and other medical professionals. Athletic trainers also spend a great deal of time counseling student athletes on the importance of proper diet, exercise, and rest, as well as the dangers of performance-enhancing drugs.

Athletic trainers also work outside of the athletic arena. They develop athletic training programs for professional and amateur dancers, cheerleaders, and other entertainers. Some of the entertainment venues and performing arts groups that have such programs include Disney World, Cirque du Soleil, the Pittsburgh Ballet Theater, and Blue Man Group.

Offices of physicians employ athletic trainers to handle some of the duties of physicians, such as taking patient histories, offering tips on exercise and nutrition, and developing rehabilitation plans for patients with injuries.

Athletic trainers in industrial and occupational settings help workers avoid or reduce the chance of injury. If a worker is injured, athletic trainers develop rehabilitation plans that seek to return the individual to work as quickly as possible.

Fire and police academies employ athletic trainers to keep recruits healthy, provide education about proper nutrition and exercise techniques, and help restore recruits to health if they become injured or ill.

Work schedules for full-time athletic trainers vary depending upon their work settings. Athletic trainers working for athletic organizations will have longer hours when their particular sport is in season—70- to 80-hour weeks are the average. They will also be scheduled to work in the evenings and on weekends, and they must be flexible if games or practices are cancelled and rescheduled. While shorter hours are typical in the off-season, athletic trainers are still in demand for training and conditioning sessions. They work indoors in training or exercise rooms and in stadiums and practice areas, as well as outdoors on athletic fields.

Athletic trainers working in a health care setting such as a hospital or rehabilitation center can expect to work regular hours, about 40 hours a week. They primarily work indoors.

REQUIREMENTS

HIGH SCHOOL

Take as many physical education and health classes as possible in high school. Anatomy and physiology courses will help you understand the human body. English and speech classes will help you to learn how to communicate effectively with coworkers, administrators, athletes, and clients. You should also take first-aid and CPR classes if they are offered.

POSTSECONDARY TRAINING

Athletic trainers must have at least a bachelor's degree in athletic training or a related major to work in the field. The National Athletic Trainers' Association (NATA) reports that nearly 70 percent of trainers who are certified by the organization have a master's degree or higher. Degrees are typically in athletic training, education, exercise physiology, wellness and health promotion, or counseling. A master's degree may be required for some managerial positions and jobs at colleges and universities.

The Commission on Accreditation of Athletic Training Education (www.caate.net) accredits athletic training programs. According to NATA, students receive instruction in the following topics in an accredited athletic training education program: Basic and Applied Sciences (human anatomy and physiology, biology, statistics and research design, exercise physiology, kinesiology/biomechanics, chemistry, and physics) and Professional Content (risk management and injury prevention, pathology of injuries and illnesses, orthopedic clinical examination and diagnosis, medical conditions and disabilities, acute care of injuries and illnesses, therapeutic modalities, conditioning, rehabilitation exercise and referral, pharmacology, psychosocial intervention and referral, nutritional aspects of injuries and illnesses, and health care administration).

CERTIFICATION AND LICENSING

Athletic trainers who have at least a bachelor's degree and pass an examination can become certified by the Board of Certification (www.bocatc.org). Those who complete these requirements can use the designation, athletic trainer-certified. The work of athletic trainers is licensed or otherwise regulated in 47 states (except Alaska, California, West Virginia, and the District of Columbia). One major licensing requirement is certification from the Board of Certification. Contact your state's department of regulation for information on requirements in your state.

OTHER REQUIREMENTS

Athletic trainers need good interpersonal and communication skills because they deal with a wide variety of people in the course of their typical work day. At one point they may talk with a football player about knee pain he is experiencing. They will then consult with the team physician regarding the player's health complaint to determine if diagnostic tests are needed or to develop a course of treatment to address this issue. At another time, they may be required to meet with administrators to review offseason conditioning plans for the soccer team or discuss department budgets.

Trainers should be in good physical condition. They frequently work long hours and may be required to stand for significant periods of time. Trainers also frequently walk, run, stoop, kneel, reach, or crawl in the course of their work.

Other important traits for athletic trainers include a strong desire to help others, good organizational skills, the ability to make quick decisions under pressure (especially when an athlete is injured), good time-management skills, and a willingness to continue to learn throughout their careers.

EXPLORING

There are many ways to learn more about a career as an athletic trainer. You can read books and magazines about the field, visit the websites of college athletic training programs to learn about typical classes and possible career paths, and ask your teacher or school counselor to arrange an information interview with an athletic trainer. Professional associations can also provide information about the field. The National Athletic Trainers' Association provides a wealth of information at its website, www.nata.org. You should also try to land a part-time job with an organization that employs athletic trainers. This will give you a chance to interact with trainers and see if the career is a good fit for your abilities and interests.

EMPLOYERS

Approximately 26,000 athletic trainers are members of the National Athletic Trainers' Association. They are employed by schools at all levels; athletic training facilities; hospitals; amateur, professional, and Olympic sports venues; clinics; offices of physicians and other health care professionals; community facilities; government agencies; workplaces; and the U.S. military.

GETTING A JOB

Many athletic trainers obtain their first jobs as a result of contacts made through college internships, career fairs, or networking events. Others seek assistance in obtaining job leads from college career services offices, newspaper want ads, and employment websites. Additionally, the National Athletic Trainers' Association provides job listings at its website, www.nata.org/career-center. Those interested in positions with the federal government should visit the U.S. Office of Personnel Management's website, www.usajobs.opm.gov.

ADVANCEMENT

There are not too many ways for athletic trainers to advance unless they pursue additional education. Athletic trainers advance by receiving pay raises and/or by taking on managerial duties (becoming head trainer, sometimes also called the director of sports medicine), or by working for higher-profile employers (such as moving from work as an athletic trainer for a college team to the same position with a professional team). With advanced education, athletic trainers can become athletic directors, team physicians, or college professors. Some go into sports equipment sales and marketing.

EARNINGS

Salaries for athletic trainers vary by type of employer, geographic region, and the worker's experience, education, and skill level. Median annual salaries for athletic trainers were $41,340 in 2009, according to the U.S. Department of Labor (USDL). Salaries ranged from less than $25,510 to $65,140 or more. The USDL reports the following mean annual earnings for athletic trainers by employer: spectator sports, $54,710; elementary and secondary schools, $52,090; colleges, universities, and professional schools, $44,250; general medical and surgical hospitals, $42,620; offices of other health care practitioners, $40,220; and other amusement and recreation industries, $40,090.

Employers offer a variety of benefits to full-time athletic trainers, including the following: medical, dental, and life insurance; paid holidays, vacations, and sick and personal days; 401(k) plans; profit-sharing plans; retirement and pension plans; and reimbursement for education required to maintain one's certification. Self-employed athletic trainers must provide their own benefits.

EMPLOYMENT OUTLOOK

Employment for athletic trainers is expected to grow much faster than the average for all careers through 2018, according to the U.S. Department of

Labor. Opportunities should be especially strong in high schools and the health care industry. New jobs will also be available in fitness and recreation sports centers and elementary schools. There will be stronger competition for jobs with college and professional sports teams.

FOR MORE INFORMATION

For information on accredited athletic training programs and careers, contact **National Athletic Trainers' Association** 2952 Stemmons Freeway Dallas, TX 75247-6113 214-637-6282 www.nata.org

Interview: Sue Stanley-Green

The editors of *Hot Health Care Careers* discussed the field of athletic training with Sue Stanley-Green, M.S., ATC, LAT, who has worked in the field for more than 30 years. For most of her professional life, Sue worked at the collegiate level as an athletic trainer. For the last 12 years, she has been an athletic training education program director and professor at Florida Southern College. She is also a member of the National Athletic Trainers' Association Hall of Fame.

Q.   What made you want to enter this career?

A.   I started in athletic training accidentally. I had never heard of an athletic trainer when I went to college. I was at Ohio State University, and a friend of mine was meeting with the head football athletic trainer. I went along because we got to enter a closed football practice, and I thought that was very cool. While I was there I figured I should ask about a career for a female in athletic training. He introduced me to Linda Daniel, the co-head athletic trainer at Ohio State in charge of the women's sports. Linda was one of the first women in the field, and I was so impressed with her. I observed the athletic trainers and what they did, and I was hooked! It was that combination of medicine and sports that I didn't know existed. I never considered another profession after that day.

Q.   What is one thing that young people may not know about a career in athletic training?

A.   Many people don't know that athletic trainers can work in many settings. We traditionally work at a high school, a college, or in professional sports. Athletic trainers also work in a clinic, with the performing arts like Cirque du Soleil or the Rockettes, or with a ballet company. They can work with the military, with new recruits or with the Navy Seals and Special Forces. Astronauts or people who work in a factory may be our patients. You can match the job setting with the type of lifestyle you would like to have. Our athletic training students are currently working with a range of athletes at Florida Southern College and from a variety of professions—from SWAT team snipers to violin players.

Q. Can you describe a day in your life on the job?

A. My life as an athletic training professor is very different from my former life in the athletic training room. My hours are much better now! In my former life, I worked at a Division I university. I was usually at work by 7:00 A.M. We saw all of our injured athletes between 7:00 and 8:00 A.M. so the coaches could have an injury report to plan for practice or games. We did most of our administrative work in the morning and treated and rehabilitated athletes between their classes. At about 1:00 the athletes started piling in the doors to be treated, taped, wrapped, and braced before practice. I worked with the football team, so I hit the field when they did. With a staff of athletic training students, graduate assistants, and full-time athletic trainers, we covered all the sports practices and were ready for anything——from the minor sprain, strain, or contusion to a major head/neck injury or heat illness. After practice, we treated the wounded; set physician appointments, x-rays, or MRIs for the next day; and completed a lot of necessary paperwork. I attended most of the home events of all of our sports to help and support our other athletic training staff members. During the season we also traveled to the away games. Road trips were fun, but they included packing for the trip and planning for meals and snacks for the players along with other adminis-trative duties. We worked seven days a week. On Sundays, we usually had treatments for a couple of hours, so it was an easy day.

As an athletic training education program director, I am at work by 8:30 and teach class most of the morning. In the afternoons, I prepare for classes, grade papers and tests, go to meetings, meet with students, assist in the athletic training room, and visit some of our clinical sites. I usually try to leave by 5:00 to pick up my daughter. I always take work home with me. I don't work too many weekends, and I am on a nine-month contract. I come to work a lot in the summer just to get ready for the next academic year. There are always lots of changes in academics to keep up on. I like the environment of being around college-aged stu-dents and student athletes. Athletic trainers and coaches are my favorite people. They tend to be positive, upbeat, and very funny. Having a sense of humor in athletic training is absolutely a requirement.

Q. What are some of the pros and cons of your job?

A. The "pros" are definitely the relationships you build with your col-leagues, students, athletes, coaches, and staff. Even 20 years later, I stay in touch with many of the people who touched and enriched my life in the world of athletics. My best and forever friends are fellow athletic trainers. I am also married to an athletic trainer, and we have worked together most of our professional lives. My husband's motto for athletic training is "Memories, Friends, and 8 x 10's,"and that is very true.

The "cons" are the hours you have to devote to the job and the lack of control in your life. If you work in a traditional setting with a team, your schedule may change because of practice facility limitations. You may practice after a game because your coach wants to make a point to the team. You may have plans for dinner and a concert, but instead you find yourself sitting in an emergency room with an athlete who sus-tained a serious injury. There is usually flexibility in our schedules dur-ing the day, but the days are often very long.

Q. What advice would you give to young people who are interested in the field?

A. Because I am the program director in an athletic training education program, I give advice to young people every day! Just ask them! The one thing I tell them daily is to be the best you can be. There are plenty of mediocre athletic trainers in our profession. Don't be mediocre! This is a decision you can make. Do you want to be good, or do you want to be great? Decide to work hard, learn everything you can, get involved, meet every athletic trainer you can, and practice your skills. I recommend getting involved in the National Athletic Trainers' Association at the state, district, or national level. I believe one should always give back to one's profession. I have experienced so many incredible things because of athletic training. I have traveled all over the world with teams. I have met so many amazing people because of being an athletic trainer. My life has never been boring or dull.

Q. What is the employment outlook for athletic trainers? How is the field changing?

A. I believe we are still exploring opportunities for athletic trainers. There are so many practice settings that were not in existence when I came out of school. I believe the one thing that sets us aside from other professions is our association with sports. We are the ones who evaluate and care for the athletes on the field, refer them if necessary, treat their injury or condition, rehabilitate them, and then return them to play. The other practice settings follow the athletic model. What makes us unique is being involved from the moment of injury until the return to play. That creates the bond with the athlete that makes this profession so special and so rewarding.

The field is changing because we are recognized as a medical profession and we are starting to get the respect we deserve. People realize if we treat people with musculoskeletal injuries immediately and aggressively like we treat athletes, they get better more quickly and can return to what they want to do. Our theory of care is starting to benefit other people than just those that play on a field or court. It is an exciting time for athletic training.

Interview: Brian Robinson

Brian Robinson, M.S., ATC, LAT is the head athletic trainer at Glenbrook South High School in Glenview, Illinois. He has been an athletic trainer for more than 30 years. He discussed his career with the editors of *Hot Health Care Careers*.

Q. Please briefly describe a day in your life on the job. What is your work environment like?

A. I am the head athletic trainer for a suburban Chicago high school with a student population of 2,800. Approximately 60 percent of our students are involved in interscholastic sports. We offer 28 sports for boys and girls. There are three to five levels of each sport, including a Frosh A and Frosh B teams, sophomore teams, junior varsity teams, and varsity teams. This spring we have nearly 1,000 students participating in athletics. During the school year, my day starts at 10 A.M. unless there is a special need for me to arrive earlier. I am available during the school day to evaluate, diagnose, treat, and rehabilitate athletic injuries. We are fortunate in Illinois to require that high school students participate in physical education classes every day for all four years of high school. If a student cannot participate due to an injury, we can work with that student in conjunction with his or her physician to provide treatment and rehabilitation during his or her scheduled physical education class. This obviously benefits the student, his or her parents, and the local physicians applaud this service, since they know their patients are receiving daily treatment for their injuries. I am fortunate to have two highly qualified certified athletic trainers working with me as well. The intensity picks up after school as we evaluate and treat athletes before their practices or games. We are on campus to provide comprehensive athletic health care to any athlete who may be injured during that afternoon or evening's practices or contests. If there are no contests scheduled for that day, we may end our day at 8 P.M. If there are contests that afternoon or evening, we may not leave the athletic training room until midnight.

We have a well-equipped athletic training room with a variety of electrical modalities as well as hydrotherapy equipment. In addition, we have various forms of strength and cardiovascular equipment to help us return the athlete to competition. We utilize this equipment to enhance the healing and rehabilitative process of our student-athletes. We also utilize our vast knowledge of functional exercises to help our students prevent injuries and return to full participation hopefully stronger than they were before the injury. We accompany teams to our various practice and contest facilities to observe our students returning from injury as well as to deal with any emergency situation that may arise. We spend a great deal of time analyzing the functional status of our recuperating athletes.

My immediate supervisor is the director of athletics at our school. I work in close contact with the physicians and families of our injured student-athletes. In most cases, high schools have limited resources for this type of program, therefore the athletic trainer must be very creative in not only obtaining the necessary equipment, but also in designing alternative methods of getting his or her athletes back to competition. Many high schools do not have the top-of-the-line rehabilitative or strength equipment available, so the athletic trainer relies on his or her creativity using stretch bands, milk jugs filled with sand, or horse troughs filled with ice water for reducing swelling in injured limbs and rehabilitating injuries.

Q. **What are the most important personal and professional qualities for people in your career?**

A. One of the most important qualities is patience, especially with the age group we deal with here, the teenaged student-athlete. Communication is the key element when speaking with parents, students, coaches, physicians, and administrators. There are hundreds of interactions every day with different people. Professional appearance is also important. There is a great deal of truth in the statement, "You only have one chance to make a first impression." Obviously compassion is a necessary trait. You are dealing with an impressionable age group as well as with parents who have a huge investment in their children. Listening skills as well as problem solving are integral skills one must possess in order to successfully diagnose athletic-related injuries.

Q. What are some of the pros and cons of your job?

A. The greatest thrill I get from this profession is the opportunity to help someone every day. The sense of accomplishment you feel when you help someone get back to the sport he or she loves after an injury that has left him or her watching from the sidelines is most gratifying. The chance to make a difference in someone's life is not something that everyone has the chance to experience.

The hours are long. This is not a 9-5 job, never was, never will be. If a person is looking for regular hours, this is not the profession for them. There are many 12- to 15-hour days. Rare is the typical 40-hour work week. There are many early morning treatment times as well as late-night games or practices. Saturday hours are frequent. Stress levels can increase when dealing with unhappy athletes, frustrated coaches, and overbearing parents. Although I am fortunate to have a well-paying position, I do hear the complaint that the field does not pay well. I really think that varies by geography and setting. It is paramount that athletic trainers working in the secondary-school setting learn to quantify their value. Since we do not generate revenue for the school, this can be difficult, but it is possible.

Q. What is the future employment outlook for athletic trainers? How is the field changing?

A. The secondary-school setting has the greatest room for growth. Only approximately 42 percent of the public high schools in the country have the services of a certified athletic trainer. There are more than 10,000 high schools without an athletic trainer to create an athletic health care program for their students.

Whereas in the past, it has been commonplace for secondary-school administrators to declare that they cannot afford the services of an athletic trainer, in today's litigious society they are finding that they cannot afford to NOT have the services of an athletic trainer. Unfortunately, an increasing number of school districts have discovered this financial reality the hard way. The athletic trainer is being recognized as a critical component of any secondary-school risk management program. The relatively small expenditure for salary and benefits allotted to an athletic trainer may prevent a multimillion-dollar settlement against a school district for an injury related to interscholastic athletics.

As the population grows older, but continues to remain active, an increasing number of people are gaining exposure to the profession of athletic training. Parents who benefited from the services of an athletic trainer either in college or in high school are now seeking high school athletic programs that employ the expertise of the athletic trainer, so their children may also benefit from these professionals. The profession is expanding into the area of working with the military as well as the "industrial athlete." Companies such as Delta Airlines employ athletic trainers to provide wellness programs and rehabilitation programs for their employees at a tremendous cost savings with regards to insurance outlays.

BIOMEDICAL ENGINEERS

OVERVIEW

Biomedical engineers use their knowledge of engineering principles and medical and biological science to improve medical instrumentation, equipment, and products; health management and care delivery systems; and medical information systems. Their work has led to important medical developments such as artificial limbs, magnetic imaging equipment, and pharmaceuticals. A minimum of a bachelor's degree in biomedical engineering, along with secondary study in another engineering discipline (such as mechanical engineering), is needed to enter the field. Approximately 16,000 biomedical engineers are employed in the United States. Employment for biomedical engineers is expected to be excellent through 2018.

THE JOB

If you have certain vision problems, you can wear disposable contact lenses to correct your vision. If you suffer from heart failure, you may be a candidate to receive an artificial heart transplant. If you recently lost a tooth, your dentist may recommend a dental implant. If you are injured during a football game, an x-ray may be ordered to rule out any fractures. As a child, you received important immunizations to guard against potentially deadly childhood diseases. What do all these situations have in common? These procedures and treatments were made possible through the work of biomedical engineers.

Biomedical engineering is a field that combines the problem-solving techniques and analytical principles of engineering with medical and biological sciences in order to help improve the diagnosis and delivery of health care.

Many biomedical engineers are involved in the research and development of medical devices that help diagnose diseases or conditions, and they develop technology that can cure, treat, or prevent diseases. Many patients owe their quality of life, if not their actual lives, to the implantation of artificial organs such as hearts, pacemakers, and cochlear implants. These devices are self supporting, and they function without a stationary power supply. Other devices currently in various stages of research and development include a bio-artificial liver and an artificial lung.

Biomedical engineers are also responsible for many devices, which, while needing continuous power supply, filtering, or chemical processing, are critically important in providing life support. An example of such a device is a dialysis machine, which improves the quality of life for people with diabetes.

Biomedical engineers also design various prostheses—artificial body parts that replace real ones. Artificial hip and knee implants help many elderly patients escape the pain caused by age or chronic diseases such as arthritis. People who have lost arms and legs due to injury or disease can increase their mobility with robotic prostheses.

Delivery of health care treatment is also improved due to the work of biomedical engineers. Tools developed by engineers range from the familiar—latex gloves, wheelchairs, tongue depressors, bedpans, and adhesive bandages—to the highly specialized, such as laser surgical tools and instruments. Think of what your next hospital procedure or doctor's visit would be like without these items!

Some biomedical engineers specialize in the design and development of biotherapies and biotechnologies. These projects include pharmaceuticals and immunizations. Biotechnology improvements include tissue engineering in the form of artificial skin embedded in collagen, which is used for skin grafts; human-made insulin, to help regulate diabetes; and the development of laboratory-generated bone substitute, to replace human bones lost due to injury or disease.

Biomedical engineers also adapt computer software or hardware to create various health care applications. Medical imaging equipment includes 2D or 3D x-rays, magnetic resonance imaging instruments, and nuclear imaging equipment, such as positron emission tomography. These systems allow physicians to diagnose an injury or disease or to identify the location of tumors or other abnormalities. Computer applications can also help guide medical procedures such as angioplasty.

Some biomedical engineers develop computerized models to help teach students about bodily functions and systems. For example, a model of the human circulatory system is often used for teaching purposes in classrooms and museums.

Biomedical engineers do not come up with these advancements and technologies overnight. Rather, they are the result of years of research, testing, and more testing—regardless of the size or scope of the project. First the need for the application or project is identified. For example, when developing the artificial heart, the medical community expressed the need for such a device in order to lower the number of heart transplant procedures, considering the demand far exceeded the supply. Working with the design and functions of available heart-lung machines at the time, biomedical engineers along with physicians went through several drafts of artificial heart designs. The first few hearts were implanted in many test animals before the first clinical trial could be conducted on a human. Throughout the testing, approval was sought in the United States, and it was finally granted by the Food and Drug Administration. Much additional research, more redesigning, and more testing were done to the prototype before the artificial heart reached the type used in surgical procedures today. Biomedical engineers are constantly improving the design, quality, and durability of artificial hearts due to changing research and technology.

In addition to their laboratory duties, some biomedical engineers supervise technicians and laboratory assistants. They present their research to the medical community, government agencies, or private companies. Some biomedical engineers teach at the university level.

Biomedical engineers have a variety of work environments depending on their employer. However, they typically work indoors in comfortable, well-lit offices and laboratories. Full-time biomedical engineers typically work 40 hours a week, but they often work longer hours as deadlines approach or if assigned an urgent project. They often travel from laboratory to laboratory or to meet with other specialists working on a project.

REQUIREMENTS

HIGH SCHOOL

In high school, take as many courses as possible in the life sciences, such as biology, anatomy and physiology, and chemistry. Other useful classes include English, mathematics, drafting, shop, computer science, speech, and health.

POSTSECONDARY TRAINING

You will need a minimum of a bachelor's degree in biomedical engineering, along with secondary study in another engineering discipline (such as electronics or mechanical engineering), to enter the field. Another option is to earn a bachelor's degree in electrical, chemical, or mechanical engineering with a specialty in biomedical engineering. Engineers who work in research laboratories typically need a graduate degree. The Accreditation Board for Engineering and Technology (ABET) accredits biomedical engineering programs. Visit its website, www.abet.org, to access a database of accredited programs in the United States.

CERTIFICATION AND LICENSING

Engineers whose work affects property, health, or life must be licensed as professional engineers. According to the U.S. Department of Labor, "this licensure generally requires a degree from an ABET-accredited engineering program, four years of relevant work experience, and completion of a state examination. Recent graduates can start the licensing process by taking the examination in two stages. The initial Fundamentals of Engineering examination can be taken upon graduation. Engineers who pass this examination commonly are called engineers in training (EITs) or engineer interns. After acquiring suitable work experience, EITs can take the second examination, called the Principles and Practice of Engineering exam." Visit the National Council of Examiners for Engineering and Surveying website, www.ncees.org, for more information on licensure.

OTHER REQUIREMENTS

Communication skills are important, since biomedical engineers often meet with other members of a design team or with other health care professionals. They must be able to explain the goals and scientific framework of their project to other engineers, medical professionals, and laypeople. At times the job is quite stressful and demanding, especially when working with an extremely complicated design or system, or when faced with tedious testing and retesting of a product. Successful biomedical engineers are calm and focused, even during the most demanding of situations. Other important traits include an analytical personality, the ability to solve problems, and scientific ability.

Did You Know?

The field of biomedical engineering has the highest number of female engineers in any engineering discipline. According to the American Society for Engineering Education, 43.7 percent of biomedical engineering students are women.

EXPLORING

There are many ways to learn more about a career as a biomedical engineer. You can read books and magazines about the field, attend an afterschool or summer engineering program (see www.careercornerstone.org/pcsumcamps.htm for more information), and join the Junior Engineering Technical Society. Ask your teacher or school counselor to arrange an information interview with a biomedical engineer. Visit the websites of college biomedical engineering programs to learn about typical classes and possible career paths. Professional associations can also provide information about the field. The Biomedical Engineering Society offers several useful resources at its website (www.bmes.org), including an electronic brochure, *Planning a Career in Biomedical Engineering,* and information on its high school programs.

EMPLOYERS

Approximately 16,000 biomedical engineers are employed in the United States. They work for colleges and universities, hospitals, research facilities, pharmaceutical companies, and government agencies.

GETTING A JOB

Many biomedical engineers obtain their first jobs as a result of contacts made through college internships, career fairs, or networking events. Others seek assistance in obtaining job leads from college career services offices, newspaper want ads, and employment websites. Additionally, professional associations, such as the Biomedical Engineering Society, provide job listings at their websites. See For More Information for a list of organizations. Those interested in positions with the federal government should visit the U.S. Office of Personnel Management's website, www.usajobs.opm.gov.

ADVANCEMENT

Biomedical engineers who are employed in nonacademic settings advance by receiving pay raises and supervisory duties, by working on more prestigious projects, and by receiving additional grant money to work on research projects. Those who work at colleges and universities as educators advance from the position of instructor, to assistant professor, to associate professor, and finally to professor—with an overall goal of attaining tenure. According to the U.S. Department of Labor, "tenured professors cannot be fired without just cause and due process." Once a professor is tenured, he or she might advance by serving as department head or becoming a dean or even college president.

Some biomedical engineers use their bachelor's degree in biomedical engineering as a first step toward attending graduate or medical school and pursuing careers in law, business, medicine, dentistry, or veterinary science.

EARNINGS

Starting salaries for bioengineering and biomedical engineering graduates with a bachelor's degree averaged $54,158 in July 2009, according to the National Association of Colleges and Employers.

Median annual salaries for biomedical engineers were $78,860 in 2009, according to the U.S. Department of Labor (USDL). Salaries ranged from less than $49,480 to $123,270 or more. The USDL reports the following mean annual earnings for biomedical engineers by employer: navigational, measuring, electromedical, and control instruments manufacturing, $92,330; scientific research and development services, $86,150; medical equipment and supplies manufacturing, $81,590; pharmaceutical and medicine manufacturing, $81,150; and general medical and surgical hospitals, $66,250.

Employers offer a variety of benefits, including the following: medical, dental, and life insurance; paid holidays, vacations, and sick and personal days; 401(k) plans; profit-sharing plans; retirement and pension plans; and educational-assistance programs. Self-employed workers must provide their own benefits.

EMPLOYMENT OUTLOOK

Employment for biomedical engineers is expected to be excellent through 2018, according to the U.S. Department of Labor. In fact, employment is expected to grow by 72 percent from 2008 to 2018. The growing and aging U.S. population and demand for new medical devices and equipment is creating strong demand for biomedical engineers. Opportunities will be particularly good in pharmaceutical manufacturing and related industries.

FOR MORE INFORMATION

Visit the institute's website for a glossary of biomedical engineering terms.
American Institute for Medical and Biological Engineering
1701 K Street, NW, Suite 510
Washington, DC 20036-1520
www.aimbe.org

To learn more about engineering education and publications, contact
American Society for Engineering Education
1818 N Street, NW, Suite 600
Washington, DC 20036-2479
www.asee.org

To read *Planning a Career in Biomedical Engineering,* visit the following Web site
Biomedical Engineering Society
8201 Corporate Drive, Suite 1125
Landover, MD 20785-2224
www.bmes.org

For career information, contact
Biotechnology Industry Organization
1201 Maryland Avenue, SW, Suite 900
Washington, DC 20024-2149
info@bio.org
www.bio.org

For information on biomedical engineering and competitions and other activities for high school students, contact
Junior Engineering Technical Society
1420 King Street, Suite 405
Alexandria, VA 22314-2750
703-548-5387
info@jets.org
www.jets.org

For a variety of information about biomedical engineering, contact
BMETnet: The Biomedical Engineering Network
www.bmenet.org

Interview: Kristina Ropella

Dr. Kristina Ropella is a professor and chair of the Department of Biomedical Engineering at Marquette University in Milwaukee, Wisconsin. She discussed her career and Marquette's program with the editors of *Hot Health Care Careers*.

Q.   What made you want to become a biomedical engineer?

A.   I was planning to attend medical school and eventually become a physician. I needed an undergraduate major. I considered several in the areas of math and science, but I chose biomedical engineering because it was a relatively new field that combined medicine with math and science, and it was interdisciplinary, requiring mastery of several disciplines in which I was interested: applied math, medicine, biology, chemistry, and physics. As I approached the end of college and worked through several internship experiences, I found that I really enjoyed the engineering and problem solving and developing technology for medical applications. I found that I was more interested in working side by side with physicians to develop new technologies for improved health care than I was interested in the day-to-day patient care.

Q.   What do you like most and least about your career?

A.   I love the interdisciplinary nature of the work and the ability to work with experts from multiple fields to solve problems. I like the ability to affect health care and improve the way we diagnose and treat health problems. As a professor, I love teaching the next generation of engineers. As a department chair, I least like the bureaucracy, paperwork, and documentation that goes along with having to run a department.

Q.   What is one thing that young people may not know about a career in biomedical engineering?

A.   It is a great springboard to so many other careers besides more traditional engineering practice. With a biomedical engineering degree, one may pursue careers in medicine, law, dentistry, education, physical therapy, hospital administration, marketing and sales of medical devices/pharmaceuticals, and more. The degree opens many doors to many careers.

Q.   Can you please tell us about your program?

A.   The Biomedical Engineering program at Marquette University is housed within the College of Engineering. We offer the B.S. degree in biomedical engineering, with majors in bioelectronics, biomechanics, and biocomputing, as well as the M.S. and Ph.D. in biomedical engineering. We also have an M.S. program in health care technologies management. We currently have 295 undergraduates and about 90 graduate students. Our graduate program has been in existence since the late 1960s, and our undergraduate program began in the early 1970s, with ABET accreditation since 1978. All pre-med/pre-dent requirements are built into our undergraduate program. We offer a cooperative education program that allows students to alternate semesters of work with semesters of school during their junior and senior years of study. Thus, the co-op participants gain at least a full-year of practical experience before graduating. We also have a strong internship program, including a special program, known as the Les Aspin Internship program, that allows students to live in Washington, D.C., and work in Food and Drug Administration laboratories during the summer or school year. Seventy-five percent of our students co-op or intern with a medical device/pharmaceutical company by the time they graduate, and more than 23 companies partner with us for co-op/internship employment. We also offer undergraduate research experiences that allow our students to work in faculty research laboratories. Our faculty and students collaborate with researchers and clinicians at the Medical College of Wisconsin, the Zablocki Veterans Administration Hospital, the Shriner's Hospital for Children-Chicago, and the Rehabilitation Institute of Chicago. These institutions provide our faculty and students with access to medical clinics, physicians, patients, other medical personnel as well as facilities and equipment used for research purposes.

Q.   What types of students pursue study in your program?

A.   We tend to have students who are talented in math and science but want to make a difference in medicine. Our students tend to be well rounded in their academic interests, often wanting more breadth in their education as opposed to too much specialization. This breadth of education also includes the arts and humanities, not just the math and sciences. Our students tend to have strong communication and leadership skills. They tend to be service oriented, wanting to be men and women for others. They are hard working, welcome a challenge, have strong moral and ethical character, and want to be leaders.

Q. **What advice would you offer biomedical engineering majors as they graduate and look for jobs?**

A. Be open to different types of job opportunities. While that first job may not be exactly what you are looking for, it will offer you great experiences and acquisition of skills that will position you to be competitive for the next career opportunity. If you talk to most people who have been working 15-20 years, they will tell you that they never imagined they would be doing the job they are today. Most of us did not plan to be in the positions we are today. We took opportunities as they came along, we took risks, stretched ourselves beyond our comfort zones, navigated uncharted territory, and ended up creating careers that fit our talents, interests, strengths, weaknesses, etc. You have quite a bit of flexibility to sculpt a career that is right for you (and your family if you choose to have one, as well), but you will have to continually assess where you are at and where you want to be, and take advantage of choices as they are presented, whether or not they were in your plans..

Q. **What is the employment outlook for biomedical engineers? Have certain areas of this field been especially promising in recent years?**

A. According to a number of indicators, like the U.S. Department of Labor, the employment outlook for biomedical engineering is strong. With a large, aging population that will require new, innovative health care technologies (including home health care) and the ongoing challenges with affordable, accessible and effective health care, the need for engineers who can solve these problems is greater than ever. Some promising (and expanding) fields include implantable devices (on the scale of nanotechnology), targeted drug delivery, medical and biological imaging, cellular and molecular engineering, systems biology, brain-machine interfaces and high-tech prosthetic devices, electronic therapy for the brain and nervous system, home health care delivery systems, and more effective delivery of vaccines/medicine in developing countries.

Interview: Nadeen Chahine

Dr. Nadeen Chahine is an assistant investigator at the Feinstein Institute for Medical Research in Manhasset, New York, and is the director of the Biomechanics & Bioengineering Laboratory. She has worked in the field for approximately 10 years. Nadeen discussed her career with the editors of *Hot Health Care Careers*.

Q. **What made you want to enter this career?**

A. I received my first degree in biomedical engineering 10 years ago. I decided to go to graduate school after that, but my research work during graduate school was also in biomedical engineering. I entered the field on a whim. When applying to college, I was introduced to the field by a recruiting/advertisement letter from the college I attended, explaining that biomedical engineering students can study engineering and be pre-med. These two aspects attracted me to the program, and so I enrolled in it.

Q. What is one thing that young people may not know about a career in biomedical engineering?

A. That it is a very versatile field. Biomedical engineers can work at a hospital, making sure that instrumentations work well. They can work at a biotech company, designing genetic treatments for rare diseases. They can work at a pharmaceutical company, making new bioreactors for drug production. They can work at implant companies, designing and testing spine implants. They can work on biomaterial or in research, understanding why humans get certain diseases. They can work in consulting or in teaching (at secondary and postsecondary levels), etc.

Q. Can you please describe a day in your life on the job?

A. My day-to-day life at my job has a lot of variation. I'm the head of a research lab. Most of my days start out with meeting with my research team to discuss what experiments they are working on and if there are any problems to discuss/address. At times, I participate in experiments myself, including working with cells and doing surgeries. I also read and write scientific reports, I analyze data for reports, I review inventory of our lab, and I request new purchases of items or equipment. I meet with collaborators and students to discuss their research projects/needs and to brainstorm new projects to work on. At times, my work requires travel to conferences or other universities/labs to present new research findings to the community.

Q. What are the most important qualities for people in your career?

A. Most important: being hard working, dedicated, smart, and creative, as well as paying attention to detail.

Q. What do you like least and most about your job?

A. Most: it never gets boring. All the exciting projects and people we work with make it an exciting job EVERY DAY. There is very little monotony in this role. Least: the job is fast paced and constantly evolving. This leaves a lot of work that overflows into personal time. It's not easy to have a work/life balance in this role.

Q. Any advice for young people who are interested in the field?

A. Yes. My advice is to get a solid engineering education in order to be a successful biomedical engineer. Also, get involved in doing research as early as possible. You will be exposed to the thinking of biomedical engineers. Use these types of opportunities to learn about how different engineers work in their respective roles in the world.

Q. What are the best ways to find a job?

A. The best way to find a job is to do internships/volunteer work. This will showcase your talent and dedication to someone who may be able to hire you for a full-time job in the future.

DENTAL ASSISTANTS

OVERVIEW

Dental assistants help dentists and other members of the dental team work more efficiently by handling a variety of duties. They are responsible for some patient care, laboratory duties, and administrative duties such as assisting dentists during patient examinations and procedures, preparing casts, handing tools to dentists, and billing. Aspiring dental assistants prepare for the field by receiving on-the-job training or by earning a certificate or diploma in dental assisting at a postsecondary academic institution. Approximately 295,300 dental assistants are employed in the United States. Employment for dental assistants is expected to be excellent through 2018.

FAST FACTS

High School Subjects
  Business
  Health
Personal Skills
  Helping
  Technical
Minimum Education Level
  High school diploma
Salary Range
  $22,000 to $33,000 to
  $47,000+
Employment Outlook
  Much faster than the average
O*NET-SOC
  31-9091.00
GOE
  14.03.01
DOT
  079
NOC
  3411

THE JOB

A good dental assistant can increase the efficiency of an entire dental team, allowing its members to see more patients in a timely manner. Depending on the size of the practice, the dental assistant's role can encompass patient care and administrative and laboratory duties.

Dental assistants prepare the examination room prior to a patient's visit. They clean and sterilize equipment and tools and set up instrument trays, making sure all necessary tools and supplies are in place for the dentist and dental hygienist. When a new patient visits the office, dental assistants record his or her personal information and medical history and enter it in a computer database. They then direct the patient to the exam room and settle him or her into the chair. Some dental assistants may take patients' blood pressure and pulse. During the examination or procedure, dental assistants work alongside the dentist, handing him or her tools, providing suction, or wiping water, paste, or saliva from the patient's mouth.

After the examination, dental assistants instruct patients regarding necessary post-operative care of the mouth or any wounds. Some dental assistants are trained to remove sutures or apply local anesthetics. They give patients general oral care tips, including describing the proper way to brush and floss teeth. They often assemble and hand out oral care kits to patients after each dental visit.

Dental assistants also have laboratory duties. They may be trained to take x-rays (radiographs) of the patients' gums and teeth as well as process the x-ray films. They also prepare materials for impressions or fillings.

Depending on state regulations, dental assistants can be trained to make casts of teeth from impressions created by dentists. They clean and polish removable appliances or make temporary crowns. If the dental office offers cosmetic procedures such as ultrasonic bleaching treatments, dental assistants can be trained to prepare the patient's mouth and gums with protective wax or other substances.

Administrative duties encompass a large portion of the dental assistant's workday. Dental assistants oversee the front office, including fielding phone calls, scheduling and confirming patients' appointments, and greeting patients as they arrive. They keep careful records of patients and the treatments performed during the appointment. They may be asked to make copies of x-rays, test results, or other paperwork for patients or other dentists.

Depending on the size of the office, dental assistants may be responsible for the billing. They often consult with insurance companies or government agencies such as Medicare regarding procedure costs or patient deductibles. Dental assistants keep track of payments made, either through insurance checks or private methods. Most dental offices now bill insurance companies electronically, so dental assistants are specially trained in the ins and outs of electronic billing, including proper procedural codes.

Dental assistants also keep track of and order supplies and equipment. Some dental assistants, especially those employed at pediatric dental offices, take photographs of children after a no-cavity dental visit. In general, many dental assistants act as the dental practice's office manager.

Dental assistants work in well-lighted, clean, and comfortable offices. They often sit in the front office when conducting administrative duties. When working with patients or assisting the dental team, they often maintain a work area near the dentist's chair. Nearly half of all dental assistants work a 35-40 hour work week, with some evening and Saturday hours.

Dental assistants are required to wear gloves, masks, eyewear, and other protective clothing, especially when working with patients. Some dental assistants wear a uniform of smock and pants. Comfortable shoes are a must, since dental assistants spend much of their day on their feet, moving back and forth between exam rooms and the front office.

REQUIREMENTS

High School

Take chemistry, biology, health, speech, computer science, accounting, and business in high school to prepare for this career.

POSTSECONDARY TRAINING

Some dental assistants still learn their skills on the job, but an increasing number of dental assistants prepare for the field by completing a postsecondary dental-assisting education program that lasts nine to 11 months. Completion of this type of program typically results in a certificate or diploma. Associate's degree programs are also available. It is a good idea to attend a training program that is accredited by the Commission on Dental Accreditation (www.ada.org/267.aspx). More than 280 programs are accredited by the Commission. Once they are hired, dental assistants also complete on-the-job training to learn the specific procedures and protocols of their employer.

CERTIFICATION AND LICENSING

Dental assistants can receive the voluntary certified dental assistant (CDA) credential from the Dental Assisting National Board. The CDA is recognized or required in more than 37 states. In addition, dental assistants must be certified in cardiopulmonary resuscitation.

In some states, dental assistants must be licensed to perform expanded functions or to perform radiological procedures. Visit www.ada.org/stateorganizations.aspx for more information on certification and licensing requirements in your state.

OTHER REQUIREMENTS

Dental assistants should have a polite and calm demeanor, especially when dealing with patients in person or over the phone, or when speaking with insurance company clerks or dental supply vendors. They should be organized and work well under pressure, since a good portion of their work day is spent juggling multiple and varied tasks. Finally, they must have good manual dexterity because they need to prepare and hand a variety of instruments and materials to dentists during dental procedures.

EXPLORING

There are many ways to learn more about a career as a dental assistant. You can read books and magazines about dentistry, visit the websites of college dental-assisting programs to learn about typical classes and possible career paths, and you can ask your teacher or school counselor to arrange an information interview with a dental assistant. Professional associations can also provide information about the field. The American Dental Association provides a wealth of information on dental assistants at its website, www.ada.org/358.aspx. You should also try to land a part-time job in a dental office. This will give you a chance to interact with dental assistants and see if the career is a good fit for your interests and abilities.

EMPLOYERS

Approximately 295,300 dental assistants are employed in the United States. About 93 percent work in offices of dentists. Other employers include government agencies, the U.S. military, offices of physicians, schools and clinics (public health dentistry), hospitals, insurance companies (processing dental insurance claims), and colleges and universities (as dental educators).

GETTING A JOB

Many dental assistants obtain their first jobs as a result of contacts made through college internships, career fairs, or networking events. Others seek assistance in obtaining job leads from college career services offices, newspaper want ads, and employment websites (such as Dentalworkers.com, www.dentalworkers.com/employment). Additionally, professional dental associations provide job listings at their websites or in their publications. See For More Information for a list of organizations. Those interested in positions with the federal government should visit the U.S. Office of Personnel Management's website, www.usajobs.opm.gov.

ADVANCEMENT

Dental assistants advance by receiving pay raises and by being assigned more demanding duties—such as handling all billing for their office. With additional training, they can become office managers, dental hygienists, dental educators, or dentists. Others work in dental product sales or as insurance claims processors for dental insurance companies.

EARNINGS

Salaries for dental assistants vary by type of employer, geographic region, and the worker's experience, education, and skill level. Median annual salaries for dental assistants were $33,230 in 2009, according to the U.S. Department of Labor (USDL). Salaries ranged from less than $22,710 to $47,070 or more. The USDL reports the following mean annual earnings for dental assistants by employer: federal government, $37,690; offices of dentists, $34,010; colleges, universities, and professional schools, $33,340; and offices of physicians, $30,930.

Dental assistants usually receive benefits such as health and life insurance, vacation days, sick leave, a savings and pension plan, and an allowance for uniforms. Eighty-six percent of certified dental assistants (CDAs) received paid vacation from their employers in 2008, according to the Dental Assisting National Board. And more than 50 percent of CDAs received health benefits. Part-time workers must provide their own benefits. More than 33 percent of dental assistants work part time.

EMPLOYMENT OUTLOOK

Employment for dental assistants is expected to grow much faster than the average for all careers through 2018, according to the U.S. Department of Labor. Approximately 105,600 new positions are expected to become available from 2008 to 2018. Employment for dental assistants will be excellent as a result of several factors. The U.S. population is growing, which will create more demand for dental professionals. More middle-aged and elderly people are keeping their natural teeth, which is creating a need for more dental assistants. Finally, the overall focus on preventive dental care for people of all ages will ensure a strong employment outlook for dental professionals in coming years.

FOR MORE INFORMATION

For career information, contact
**American Dental
Assistants Association**
35 East Wacker Drive, Suite 1730
Chicago, IL 60601-2211
312-541-1550
www.dentalassistant.org

For information on dental assisting education and careers, contact
American Dental Association
211 East Chicago Avenue
Chicago, IL 60611-2678
312-440-2500
www.ada.org

For information on dental education, contact
**American Dental
Education Association**
1400 K Street, NW, Suite 1100
Washington, DC 20005-2415
202-289-7201
adea@adea.org
www.adea.org

For information about certification, contact
Dental Assisting National Board
444 North Michigan Avenue,
Suite 900
Chicago, IL 60611-3985
800-367-3262
www.dentalassisting.com

Interview: Angela M. Swatts

Angela M. Swatts, CDA, EFDA is the president of the American Dental Assistants Association. She discussed her career and the field of dental assisting with the editors of *Hot Health Care Careers*.

Q. Where do you work? How long have you worked in the field?

A. I currently manage a dental laboratory. I have been a dental assistant since 1984. I graduated from an accredited dental assisting program at the Indiana University School of Dentistry and became a CDA (certified dental assistant) in 1985.

Q. What made you want to enter this career?

A. As a child I had a lot of dentistry done as a result of an accident. I always admired the dental assistants in the office, as they were the ones responsible for making me feel safe and comfortable. I wanted to help in the same way.

Q. What is one thing that young people may not know about a career as a dental assistant?

A. The career field is very vast and wide. Once you have the basic training, you can take it as far as you want and in many directions. You can be an educator in a dental assisting program, a sales representative for a dental manufacturing company, do research, write articles, lecture, or manage a clinic.

Q. What are the most important personal and professional qualities for dental assistants?

A. First and foremost, you must be a caring individual. People put their dental health in your hands. You must be willing to continue to learn and improve your skills. Dentistry is ever changing, and you must be willing to stay current. You must be efficient.

Q. What are some of the pros and cons of your job?

A. The pros outweigh the cons by far. The hours are great, usually no nights and weekends. The people you meet over the years are fascinating. The environment is usually stress free.

Q. What advice would you give to young people who are interested in becoming dental assistants?

A. Go to an accredited program, get every possible credential, continue to learn and improve yourself, and join your professional organization.

Q. What is the employment outlook for dental assistants?

A. The outlook is great. Dentistry is not usually affected by the economy, so there is always a need for dentists and dental assistants. As access-to-care issues force states to look at ways to provide more care to the underprivileged, you will see dental assistants doing more than ever before, in order to allow the dentist to see more patients and free him or her up to handle more serious cases.

Q. How is the field changing?

A. The field is ever changing. Technology gets better, and products get better. You must stay on top of the current procedures and techniques.

Q. Can you tell us a little about the American Dental Assistants Association (ADAA)?

A. The ADAA is the oldest, largest organization representing dental assistants throughout the country and in the U.S. Army and U.S. Air Force. We supply continuing education, legislation, and membership services to more than 10,000 dental assistants.

Q. How important is association membership to career success?

A. To belong to your professional association makes a job a career. To be a professional dental assistant, you must belong to your professional organization. It is a way to stay informed and educated with regards to your profession.

DENTAL HYGIENISTS

OVERVIEW

Dental hygienists perform prophylaxis procedures on patients (preventive care that helps a patient avoid gum disease and cavities), take oral x-rays, administer local anesthetics, and remove sutures and dressings. They perform administrative duties such as charting and/ or taking oral and medical histories of patients. Dental hygienists also educate patients about the importance of oral preventive care. A minimum of an associate's degree or certificate is required to work as a dental hygienist. Approximately 174,100 dental hygienists are employed in the United States. Employment in this field is expected to grow much faster than the average for all careers through 2018.

FAST FACTS

High School Subjects
Biology
Health

Personal Skills
Helping
Technical

Minimum Education Level
Associate's degree

Salary Range
$44,000 to $67,000 to $92,000+

Employment Outlook
Much faster than the average

O*NET-SOC
29-2021.00

GOE
14.03.01

DOT
078

NOC
3222

THE JOB

Dental hygienists are licensed dental professionals who are responsible for many of the routine duties once performed by dentists—which leaves dentists free to complete more complicated and invasive procedures.

At the beginning of the appointment, the dental hygienist first assesses the patient. He or she reviews the patient's medical and oral history, takes x-rays, and conducts a clinical exam. Then he or she examines the condition of the patient's teeth as well as the periodontal area. Dental hygienists report their findings to the dentist, who then conducts a follow-up exam for a final diagnosis of any dental problems.

If the patient is there for a routine cleaning, the dental hygienist can perform the prophylaxis. This involves the removal of any tartar (hardened mineralized plaque) and stains from the surface of the teeth. Dental hygienists use various hand instruments and power-driven dental instruments to help them during the process. If the patient suffers from periodontal disease, the dental hygienist may administer a local anesthetic before continuing on with scaling (removing plaque and other stains) or root planing (more involved cleaning that focuses on the roots) to help curb the disease. The dental hygienist may also finish the session with an application of fluoride, which prevents tooth decay.

Dental hygienists may also be specially trained to remove sutures or change dressings for patients who have had oral surgery or other invasive procedures. They may also assist the dentist by creating teeth molds in preparation for denture pieces, tooth caps, or implants. They may help the dentist when providing ultrasonic teeth whitening by prepping the gum line with wax or other protective coverings.

Dental hygienists also teach patients about good oral health. They instruct the patient about the proper techniques to use when brushing and flossing their teeth. They may use a model of upper or lower teeth to demonstrate these techniques. If the patient complains of tooth sensitivity, the dental hygienist may recommend a special toothpaste or rinse to help alleviate this problem.

Depending on the size and scope of the dental office, dental hygienists may have additional duties such as charting and keeping track of and ordering necessary medical supplies.

Full-time dental hygienists work about 40 hours a week. Some evening and weekend shifts are required to accommodate patients' schedules. Dental hygienists wear professional attire, often a lab coat. Comfortable shoes are a must, since dental hygienists are on their feet for much of the day, or walking from exam room to exam room. They also wear latex gloves, masks, and other protective equipment when working with patients.

Dental hygienists work in clean, comfortable, well-lit offices. They often sit on stools when performing procedures in order to better reach the patient. Dental hygienists are at high risk of developing carpal tunnel syndrome—nerve damage to the hand caused by the use of small tools in repetitive movements. Dental hygienists often use special braces and perform stretching exercises to reduce the risk of developing carpal tunnel syndrome.

At times, dental hygienists' work schedules can be quite hectic, especially when handling a heavy patient load. They can also fall behind schedule due to a difficult case or a patient who is especially nervous or jittery. They also may work at more than one office—sometimes even in the course of a single workday. If the dental hygienist is employed at more than one facility, he or she needs a reliable means of transportation in order to travel from one office to another.

REQUIREMENTS

HIGH SCHOOL

Take courses in biology, chemistry, psychology, math, and health. Speech classes will help you develop your communication skills, which you will use often when interacting with patients, dentists, dental assistants, and other hygienists.

POSTSECONDARY TRAINING

A minimum of an associate's degree or certificate is required to work as a dental hygienist. More than 310 dental hygiene programs are accredited by the

Did You Know?

✔ According to the American Dental Hygienists' Association, the typical dental hygiene educational program requires 86 credit hours for an associate degree and 122 credit hours for a bachelor's degree.

✔ Ninety-seven percent of dental hygiene students are female.

✔ Nearly 87 percent of dental hygiene students are Caucasian.

Source: American Dental Hygienists' Association

Commission on Dental Accreditation. Visit www.ada.org/267.aspx for a list of accredited programs. Most programs award an associate's degree, but some offer certificates, bachelor's degrees, and master's degrees. According to the American Dental Hygienists' Association (ADHA), a typical associate's degree program offers courses in the basic sciences (anatomy, physiology, pathology, general chemistry, biochemistry, microbiology, pathology, nutrition, and pharmacology), the liberal arts (English, speech, sociology, and psychology), dental science courses (dental anatomy, head and neck anatomy, oral pathology, radiography, oral embryology and histology, periodontology, and pain control and dental materials), and dental hygiene science courses (patient management, clinical dental hygiene, oral health education/preventive counseling, community dental health, and medical and dental emergencies). Students also participate in preclinical and clinical experiences in which they work directly with patients under the close supervision of dental educators. The average associate's degree program requires 86 credit hours, according to the ADHA. Dental hygienists who plan to work in research, clinical practice, or teaching typically have at least a bachelor's degree.

CERTIFICATION AND LICENSING

All states require dental hygienists to be licensed. According to the U.S. Department of Labor, "nearly all states require candidates to graduate from an accredited dental hygiene school and pass both a written and clinical examination. The American Dental Association's Joint Commission on National Dental Examinations administers the written examination, which is accepted by all states and the District of Columbia. State or regional testing agencies administer the clinical examination. In addition, most states require an examination on the legal aspects of dental hygiene practice."

OTHER REQUIREMENTS

To be a successful dental hygienist, you should have excellent communication and interpersonal skills, since you will spend the majority of your workday interacting with patients, dentists, and dental assistants. You should have good manual dexterity in order to skillfully use dental instruments to conduct prophylaxis procedures. Other important traits include attention to detail, punctuality, cleanliness, and patience and compassion to deal with patients who may be fearful of undergoing dental procedures.

EXPLORING

There are many ways to learn more about a career as a dental hygienist and dentistry as a whole. You can read books and magazines about the field, visit the websites of college dental hygiene programs to learn about typical classes and possible career paths, and ask your health teacher or school counselor to arrange an information interview with a dental hygienist. Professional associations can also provide information about the field. Both the American Dental Association (www.ada.org) and the American Dental Hygienists' Association (www.adha.org/careerinfo) provide a wealth of information about dental hygiene education and careers at their websites. You should also try to land a part-time job in a dental office. This will give you a chance to interact with dental hygienists and see if the career is a good fit for your interests and abilities.

Good Advice

Caryn Loftis Solie, RDH, the president of the American Dental Hygienists' Association, offers the following advice to young people who are interested in becoming dental hygienists:

"Contact the American Dental Hygienists' Association to find local dental hygienists to meet and have the opportunity to observe dental hygienists working in various settings. Take every opportunity to expand your knowledge base in science studies but also incorporate speech, interpersonal communications, and psychology."

EMPLOYERS

Approximately 174,100 dental hygienists are employed in the United States, with nearly all working in dental offices. Others work for employment services and in physicians' offices, hospitals, nursing homes, prisons, schools, and public health clinics. Some dental hygienists work for companies that sell dental-related equipment and supplies. Opportunities are also available in the U.S. military. About 50 percent of dental hygienists work part time.

GETTING A JOB

Many dental hygienists obtain their first jobs as a result of contacts made through college internships or networking events. Others seek assistance in obtaining job leads from college career services offices, newspaper want ads, employment websites, and dental auxiliary placement services (which charge a fee for their services). Additionally, professional dental associations, such as the American Dental Association, provide job listings at their web sites. See For More Information for a list of organizations. The American Dental Hygienists' Association offers tips on career planning and résumé writing at its website, www.adha.org/careerinfo/dhcareers.htm. Those interested in positions with the federal government should visit the U.S. Office of Personnel Management's website, www.usajobs.opm.gov.

ADVANCEMENT

Dental hygienists advance by receiving salary increases or by working at larger practices. Some hygienists pursue advanced education and become dentists. Others pursue bachelor's or master's degrees in dental hygiene and work as college educators or public health researchers and educators.

EARNINGS

Salaries for dental hygienists vary by type of employer, geographic region, and the worker's experience level and skills. Median annual salaries for dental hygienists were $67,340 in 2009, according to the U.S. Department of Labor (USDL). Salaries ranged from less than $44,900 to $92,860 or more. The USDL reports the following mean annual earnings for dental hygienists by employer: offices of dentists, $68,160; employment services, $68,150; outpatient care centers, $68,100; offices of physicians, $61,740; and general medical and surgical hospitals, $57,570.

Approximately 50 percent of dental hygienists received fringe benefits in 2009, according to a survey by the American Dental Hygienists' Association. Sick leave, paid vacation, and retirement plans were the most commonly cited benefits.

EMPLOYMENT OUTLOOK

Employment for dental hygienists is expected to grow much faster than the average for all careers through 2018, according to the U.S. Department of Labor. It is one of the fastest-growing careers in the United States, with growth of 36 percent expected from 2008 to 2018. Demand will increase for dental hygienists as a result of the growth of the U.S. population, the increasing focus on preventive dental care, and a growing reliance on hygienists to perform duties that were previously handled by dentists. Competition for jobs will vary by geographic region. In some areas, there is an overabundance of hygienists, which will make finding a job more difficult.

FOR MORE INFORMATION

For information on education and careers, contact
American Dental Association
211 East Chicago Avenue
Chicago, IL 60611-2678
312-440-2500
publicinfo@ada.org
www.ada.org

For information on education, contact
American Dental Education Association
1400 K Street, NW, Suite 1100
Washington, DC 20005-2415
202-289-7201
adea@adea.org
www.adea.org

For comprehensive information about a career as a dental hygienist, contact
American Dental Hygienists' Association
444 North Michigan Avenue, Suite 3400
Chicago, IL 60611-3980
312-440-8900
mail@adha.net
www.adha.org

Interview: Caryn Loftis Solie

Caryn Loftis Solie, RDH is a dental hygienist and the president of the American Dental Hygienists' Association. She discussed her career with the editors of *Hot Health Care Careers*.

Q.   What made you want to enter this career?

A.   I was inspired by a dental hygienist I met when I worked part-time in a dental office while in high school. Her ability to provide a valuable service to her patients, have diversity in her duties, and earn a reasonable income impressed me. She was very instrumental in my decision to become a dental hygienist.

Q.   What is one thing that young people may not know about a career in dental hygiene?

A.   Dental hygienists may work in a variety of settings. Many dental hygienists provide care in a private dental office, but opportunities are also available to work in hospitals, community health centers, nursing homes, schools, prisons, and mobile clinics. Dental hygienists work in public health settings as caregivers, but also as administrators. Dental hygienists are educators in dental and dental hygiene schools. Many dental manufacturers and companies hire dental hygienists as researchers, and utilize dental hygienists in product development, sales and marketing, as education specialists, and as executives.

Q.   What are the most important qualities for people in your career?

A.   It is important to be outgoing, to genuinely like people and want to help them. Being a good communicator and motivator is very important. As in any profession the qualities of hard work, dedication, and a willingness to always be learning new things are critical to your success.

Q.   What are some of the pros and cons of your job?

A.   Pros: The gratification you have in knowing you have improved someone's health and well being is tremendous. You meet many interesting people from all walks of life and each encounter gives you more knowledge. You are continually learning as science and technology make advances.

Cons: The 50 state regulations that vary in what duties a dental hygienist can perform often can be limiting to your job satisfaction. Those same regulations may impede one in easily moving from state to state.

Q.   Can you tell me about the American Dental Hygienists' Association? How important is association membership to career success?

A.   The American Dental Hygienists Association is the organization that represents the profession of dental hygiene on the national level. Each state has a chapter and there are local chapters in most communities as well. The association works to advance the profession as a whole and to provide education and support for dental hygienists. Membership in the association is a personal choice. I found that being a member and taking the opportunities to be an active member gave me more personal confidence, improved my critical thinking and public speaking skills, and opened up new venues of employment.

Interview: Charlene Uy

Charlene Uy is a registered dental hygienist. She discussed her career with the editors of *Hot Health Care Careers*.

Q. What made you want to enter this career?

A. I was always interested in dentistry due to the amount of detail that is involved in the job. I love working with my hands and building strong relationships with people. I proactively sought out opportunities in which I could gain exposure in the dental field. I volunteered at my university's dental college, where I witnessed the positive effects that the hygiene students had on their patients. After several volunteer sessions, I found myself attracted to the preventive services offered, which led to my pursuit of becoming a dental hygienist.

Q. What is one thing that young people may not know about a career in dental hygiene?

A. I think many young people confuse the dental hygienist with the dental assistant. The dental hygienist and dental assistant are two separate occupations and involve different duties in the dental office. In order to become a dental hygienist, one must take two years of prerequisites and enter a two- to three-year dental hygiene program. There is also the option of expanding your education by obtaining a master's in dental hygiene.

Q. What are the most important personal and professional qualities for people in your career?

A. Some important personal and professional qualities for people in my career are good personal hygiene, compassion, and gentleness. Good personal hygiene is very important, especially when you are viewed as a role model for good dental hygiene. As a health care provider, it is also crucial to have compassion when taking care of people's health. Aside from compassion, gentleness is a quality that dental hygienists must have. There seem to be many people who are nervous during their dental appointment and need the assurance that they can trust the dental hygienist. Having a soft touch and painless dental cleaning will ensure that patients return for future dental cleanings and procedures.

Q. What do you like most and least about your job?

A. There are many positive sides to my job, but the one thing I value the most is the fact that I can help others improve their hygiene and overall health. My job is to prevent cavities and other related dental problems from arising. I perform preventive procedures, such as dental cleanings, fluoride, dental education, nutritional counseling, and smoking cessation. I usually like to educate my patients on how their oral health is related to their overall being, such as connections to diabetes and heart disease. The one thing I find the least appealing about my job is the muscle pain I get in my arms and back after doing dental cleanings. This occurs after long hours of work. However, there are ways to alleviate and prevent muscle pain.

Q. What advice would you give to young people who are interested in the field?

A. Shadow a dental hygienist a few times in order to get a better grasp of the profession. It is best to ask as many questions as you can in order to truly know if dental hygiene is the profession for you. I would also research the different dental hygiene programs that are offered within your community. This includes what prerequisite courses you need to take in college prior to admission in the hygiene program, the application procedure, and the course load you will be expected to take while in dental hygiene school.

Q. What is the employment outlook for your field?

A. The employment outlook for dental hygienists looks to be very promising. It is one of the fastest-growing professions in this century. Preventive care provided by dental hygienists is very important—especially during this time of economic struggle. There are many job openings, and the need is always ample.

DENTISTS

OVERVIEW

Dentists provide dental care to patients of all ages. They diagnose and treat problems with teeth and surrounding tissues and administer care to prevent future dental problems. Some dentists specialize in a particular dental field, such as orthodontics or pediatric dentistry. A doctoral degree in dentistry is required to work as a dentist. Approximately 141,900 dentists are employed in the United States. Employment opportunities for dentists should be good through 2018.

THE JOB

While many people dread a visit to the dentist, a twice-yearly visit to the dentist is important to maintain your oral health. Good dental care is becoming even more important, as medical studies have linked dental health to overall health. Dentists diagnose and treat patients of all ages with any problems dealing with teeth and surrounding tissues.

FAST FACTS

High School Subjects
Chemistry
Health

Personal Skills
Critical thinking
Helping
Technical

Minimum Education Level
Dental degree

Salary Range
$69,000 to $142,000 to $304,000+

Employment Outlook
Faster than the average

O*NET-SOC
29-1021.00, 29-1022.00, 29-1023.00, 29-1024.00

GOE
14.03.01

DOT
072

NOC
3113

When seeing a new patient, dentists may ask about the patient's medical history, including any pre-existing conditions or any medications he or she is taking. The dentist may also ask the patient if he or she is experiencing any oral pain or discomfort. The next phase of the assessment can involve an oral examination and x-rays. In some dental offices, dental hygienists and assistants handle these duties. The dentist then reviews the x-ray and double-checks the patient's mouth for cavities or other dental issues.

If the patient is there for a routine visit, the dentist may proceed with the prophylaxis, or teeth cleaning, or ask the dental hygienist to complete the procedure. Dentists can also apply fluoride treatments or sealants to protect teeth from decay.

Many times, patients see dentists for pain or discomfort due to dental caries (cavities), cracked teeth, or other oral problems. For example, when treating a patient with a cavity, the dentist will first use tools such as a sickle probe (also known as a dental explorer) to locate the cavity. Once found, the dentist can use a variety of tools—picks, probes, and drills—to remove the decay. The next step involves filling the cavity with medicine to retard decay, and finally filling the cavity with a dental restoration—usually composite resin, porcelain, or even gold. Once the filling is in place, the dentist uses a file and other tools to create a natural finish. If the decay is extensive, the dentist may be forced to file the tooth down and cover it with a crown or cap made of porcelain or gold. In these instances, dentists take measurements and make a temporary model of the crown.

Sometimes teeth are so damaged that they cannot be saved. In this case, they must be extracted before infection sets in (or gets worse) or more damage is done. When conducting an extraction, dentists may need to

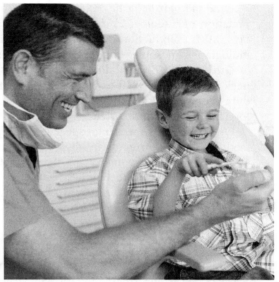

A dentist teaches a boy how to brush his teeth. (Digital Vision/Thinkstock)

administer a form of local anesthetic or even nitrous oxide to prevent the patient from feeling pain. They may also prescribe antibiotics if infection is detected.

In order to maintain optimum dental health, dentists counsel their patients on the proper way to care for their teeth. They demonstrate the correct way to brush and floss teeth and suggest special toothpastes to address issues such as tooth or gum sensitivity.

Dentists can also change the appearance of teeth through cosmetic procedures. Many patients wishing for straighter, whiter, or bigger teeth can opt for veneers, tooth bridges, bleaching, tooth reshaping, or gum lifts.

In addition to patient care, some dentists perform administrative duties. They maintain the financial records of their practice (including billing) and supervise dental hygienists, dental assistants, and other office staff.

Some dentists specialize in a particular area of dentistry. The American Dental Association recognizes nine professional specialties, which are detailed in the following paragraphs.

Dental public health specialists promote good dental health and prevent dental diseases within the community. They study the oral health needs of a community, then develop plans and policies that help community members attain better dental health.

Endodontists specialize in treating the tooth pulp and the tissues surrounding the tooth root. Endodontic procedures include root canals, endodontic retreatments, and repairing cracked teeth or other dental trauma.

Oral and maxillofacial pathologists focus on the identification and management of diseases affecting the oral and maxillofacial region—the jaws and face.

Oral and maxillofacial radiologists focus on the production and interpretation of radiological images of the oral and maxillofacial region. X-rays, MRIs, subtraction radiography, arthrography, and dental panoramic radiographs are some procedures used by these dentists.

Oral and maxillofacial surgeons operate on the mouth, jaws, teeth, gums, neck, and head, as well as the soft tissues in these regions. Some procedures done by these dental specialists include facial implants, treatments for TMJ disorder, and corrective jaw surgery.

Orthodontics is the dental specialty dealing with malocclusions of the teeth due to tooth irregularity, disproportionate jaw relationships, or both. *Orthodontists* are responsible for the correction of these malformations using procedures and techniques including expansion appliances, retainers, or fixed multi-bracket therapy—otherwise known as braces.

A Truly Unique Career

To encourage more people to become dentists, the American Dental Association (ADA) has created the following list of reasons why dentistry is "truly a unique career."

✔ **Provides the Opportunity to Provide Service to Others.** There is great personal satisfaction helping people attain better oral health. Conducting research and teaching future dentists also are rewarding.

✔ **Offers Good Balance of Professional and Personal Goals.** Approximately 75 percent of dentists are solo practitioners, which allows them to establish their own work schedules that work well with their personal lives. Most experienced dentists work a standard week of 35-40 hours—far less than the 50+ hours worked by physicians. New dentists may work longer hours as they attempt to build their practices.

✔ **Offers Strong Earning Potential.** The U.S. Census Bureau reports that salaries for dentists are among the highest 5 percent in the United States.

✔ **Prestige/Social Status.** Dentists often have strong reputations in their communities and have a "distinguished history of leadership in improving world health."

✔ **Provides Opportunities to Be Creative.** This might be surprising to some, but the ADA calls dentists "artists," who "combine keen visual memory, excellent judgment of space and shape, and a high degree of manual dexterity in the delivery of patient services."

✔ **Variety.** As mentioned earlier, there are nine dental specialties available in addition to general dentistry and a variety of employment settings that will take dentists from small towns and big cities in the United States to countries throughout the world.

Pediatric dentists specialize in the comprehensive preventive and thera-peutic oral health of infants and young children, as well as those with special needs. Pediatric dentists tailor their dental surroundings and approach to suit and soothe young children.

Periodontists specialize in the supporting and surrounding tissues of the teeth including the gums, aveola bone, cementum, and periodontal ligaments, and the diseases and conditions affecting them.

Prosthodontists replace missing teeth with permanent fixtures, such as crowns and bridges, or with removable fixtures such as dentures.

Dentists work in comfortable, well-lit offices. Many offices equip each examining room with overhead music or a television screen to keep patients occupied during examinations. All equipment and tools are sanitized and organized, and made ready for the dentists' use by trained office staff. Full-time dentists work about 36 hours a week, the majority of which are spent on patient care. Office hours may vary depending on the size of practice, and they often include Saturday and evening hours. Office attire for dentists varies from office to office but generally consists of scrubs or a medical gown. Dentists also wear gloves and masks when treating patients. Many dentists are susceptible to carpal tunnel syndrome due to repetitive movements during examinations and treatments, and continued manipulation of dental tools.

REQUIREMENTS

HIGH SCHOOL

To prepare for college, take courses in biology, organic and inorganic chemistry, mathematics, physics, computer science, and health. English and speech classes will also be useful.

POSTSECONDARY TRAINING

A doctoral degree in dentistry is required to work as a dentist. Dental students typically enter dental school after earning a bachelor's degree. Some students earn a bachelor's degree in a science-oriented field such as biology or chemistry, while others take the required science coursework while pursuing a major in a nonscientific field. Admissions requirements include strong undergraduate grades, successful completion of the Dental Admissions Test, and participation in personal interviews with dental school admissions officials. Nearly 60 dental schools in the United States are accredited by the American Dental Association's Commission on Dental Accreditation.

In recent years, the ADA has placed a strong emphasis on improving diversity among dental students. The good news: women now make up about 40 percent of dental students. The bad news: African Americans, Hispanic Americans, and Native Americans are still underrepresented in dental schools as compared to their representation in the general population, but the ADA is working hard to ensure that admission rates reflect diversity.

CERTIFICATION AND LICENSING

Dentists may obtain certification from the various dental specialty boards such as the American Board of Pediatric Dentistry and the American Board of Oral and Maxillofacial Surgery. Certification, while voluntary, is highly recommended. It is an excellent way to stand out from other dentists and demonstrate your abilities to prospective patients.

All 50 states and the District of Columbia require dentists to be licensed. Licensing requirements typically involve graduating from an accredited dental school and passing practical and written examinations. According to the U.S. Department of Labor, "candidates may fulfill the written part of the state licensing requirements by passing the National Board Dental Examinations. Individual states or regional testing agencies administer the written or practical examinations." Dental specialists must also receive special licensing. Those seeking specialty licensure must complete two to four years of postgraduate education. In some instances, applicants must also take and pass a state-level examination and complete a postgraduate residency term of up to two years.

OTHER REQUIREMENTS

Dentists need to be calm and work well under pressure, especially when working on a difficult case or with a fearful patient. Strong communication skills are also very important. Pediatric dentists often use a gentle speaking voice or rename certain tools or procedures to help calm younger patients. Other key traits for dentists include excellent manual dexterity, attentiveness to detail, diagnostic ability, and good business acumen.

EXPLORING

There are many ways to learn more about a career in dentistry. You can read books and magazines about the field, visit the websites of dental schools to learn about typical classes and possible career paths, and ask your teacher or school counselor to arrange an information interview with a dentist (or talk to your own). Professional associations can also provide information about the field. The American Dental Association provides a wealth of information on education and careers at its website, www.ada.org. You should also try to land a part-time job in a dental office. This will give you a chance to interact with dentists and see if the career is a good fit for your interests and abilities.

EMPLOYERS

Approximately 141,900 dentists are employed in the United States. About 75 percent of dentists who work in private practice are sole proprietors, and nearly 15 percent belong to a partnership. Dentists also work in many other employment settings, including those in academics as teachers, at public health facilities and hospitals, in research, and in international health care (with the World Health Organization, the Food and Agricultural Organization of the United Nations, and the United Nations

Educational, Scientific and Cultural Organization). Additionally, about 15 percent of dentists practice in dental specialties. The three largest specialties are orthodontists (7,700 people employed in this field), oral and maxillofacial surgeons (6,700), and prosthodontists (500).

GETTING A JOB

After graduation, most dental school graduates purchase an established practice or open a new practice. Dentists who do not purchase a practice or start their own business can obtain their first jobs as a result of contacts made through college internships, career fairs, or networking events. Others seek assistance in obtaining job leads from college career services offices, newspaper want ads, and employment websites (such as Dentalworkers.com, www.dentalworkers.com/employment). Those interested in positions with the federal government should visit the U.S. Office of Personnel Management's website, www.usajobs.opm.gov.

ADVANCEMENT

Dentists advance by earning higher salaries or by developing a successful practice that attracts more patients. Dentists who work as associates for established dentists may eventually start their own practice or purchase an existing practice from a dentist who is retiring or leaving the field for other reasons. Dentists also conduct research for private organizations or government agencies. Others teach dentistry at dental colleges.

EARNINGS

Salaries for general dentists vary by type of employer, geographic region, and the worker's experience. Median annual salaries for general dentists were $142,090 in 2009, according to the U.S. Department of Labor (USDL). Ten percent earned less than $69,790. The USDL reports the following mean annual earnings for general dentists by employer: state government, $150,020; outpatient care centers, $138,750; offices of physicians, $132,230; and general medical and surgical hospitals, $109,560. The American Dental Association reports that dental specialists average more than $304,000 per year.

Dentists who are salaried employees receive a variety of benefits, including the following: medical and life insurance; paid holidays, vacations, and sick and personal days; 401(k) plans; profit-sharing plans; retirement and pension plans; and reimbursement for continuing education. Self-employed dentists must provide their own benefits. Approximately 28 percent of dentists are self-employed.

EMPLOYMENT OUTLOOK

Employment for dentists is expected to grow faster than the average for all careers through 2018, according to the U.S. Department of Labor. Prospects in the specialties of orthodontics and prosthodontics are even better—with employment expected to grow much faster than the average during the same time span. More opportunities are emerging for dentists as a result of the growing U.S. population and the increasing number of people age 65 and older, who often need more dental care than other demographic groups. Other factors that are fueling growth include the increasing number of people who have dental insurance, advances in technology that are expanding treatment options, and the growing popularity of cosmetic dental procedures.

FOR MORE INFORMATION

For a wealth of information on dental education and careers, contact
American Dental Association
211 East Chicago Avenue
Chicago, IL 60611-2678
312-440-2500
publicinfo@ada.org
www.ada.org

For information on educational programs in the United States and Canada, contact
American Dental Education Association
1400 K Street, NW, Suite 1100
Washington, DC 20005-2415
adea@adea.org
www.adea.org

Contact the following organizations for more information on education and careers in dentistry:
Academy of General Dentistry
211 East Chicago Avenue, Suite 900
Chicago, IL 60611-1999
www.agd.org

American Academy of Oral & Maxillofacial Pathology
214 North Hale Street
Wheaton, IL 60187-5115
aaomp@b-online.com
www.aaomp.org

American Academy of Oral & Maxillofacial Radiology
PO Box 231422
New York, NY 10023-0024
www.aaomr.org

American Academy of Pediatric Dentistry
211 East Chicago Avenue, Suite 1700
Chicago, IL 60611-2637
312-337-2169
www.aapd.org

American Association of Endodontists
211 East Chicago Avenue, Suite 1100
Chicago, IL 60611-2691
800-872-3636
info@aae.org
www.aae.org

American Association of Orthodontists
401 North Lindbergh Boulevard
St. Louis, MO 63141-7816
info@aaortho.org
www.braces.org

American Association of Public Health Dentistry
3085 Stevenson Drive, Suite 200
Springfield, IL 62703-4270
natoff@aaphd.org
www.aaphd.org

American Association of Women Dentists
216 West Jackson Boulevard, Suite 625
Chicago, IL 60606-6945
info@aawd.org
www.aawd.org

American Student Dental Association
211 East Chicago Avenue, Suite 700
Chicago, IL 60611-2663
www.asdanet.org

Interview: Steve Morris

Dr. Steve Morris is a dentist in Chicago, Illinois. He discussed his career and the field of dentistry with the editors of *Hot Health Care Careers*.

Q. What made you want to become a dentist?

A.   I decided to become a dentist for several reasons. I worked in a pharmacy all through high school and got a chance to become acquainted with people in many areas of medicine—physicians, dentists, pharmacists, optometrists, and so on. I found of the various professions that dentistry piqued my curiosity the most. And frankly, as a child I spent quite a bit of time in the dental office, so I was very familiar with the procedures and environment. There was a kind of fascination with all the instruments and machinery. The instrumentation these days is a lot more high-tech, and it's been interesting to be able to advance as the profession does. Dentistry is a nice blend of medicine, art, and microtechnology, and it is basically all hands-on. Dentistry is also nice in that you can work in whatever setting is most appealing to you—a large group practice or small solo practice—with whatever hours work best for you.

Q. What is one thing that young people may not know about a career in dentistry?

A.   People don't always realize the many areas of dentistry that are available. There are areas to appeal to just about everyone. If you're surgically inclined, there are opportunities to do surgical reconstruction, cancer treatment, and implant dentistry. For those more artistically inclined, one can specialize in cosmetic dentistry with veneers, bonding, and orthodontics. You can work with children only with developing faces, or with the other side of the spectrum, geriatric patients with implants, dentures, or other methods of restoring lost function and esthetics. If you enjoy a little more variety, general dentists delve a bit into all the specialties and work with a wide range of age groups. There is also research and technical development, which is less patient oriented.

Q. What are the most important personal and professional qualities for dentists?

A.   There are several important qualities for dentists that will help make them happy and successful in the profession. It helps to be very patient, as some procedures can be rather time consuming and tedious, and if things don't go according to plan you have to be able to shift gears and make treatment modifications. Having good tactile sense and hand-to-eye coordination is very helpful as well. Many times procedures are accomplished by feel as much as sight, and sometimes they have to be visualized in reverse on a mirror. Practice and repetition improve these qualities, but good inherent ability makes it much easier. You have to be able to work in a small area and still be able to be pretty precise about what you're doing. Being mechanically inclined is also helpful, as many times you have to get creative and be able to use available materials for a problem you weren't expecting. You can't always prepare for what a patient will come in with, or have things go according to plan, so it pays to be flexible. You have to be even tempered enough to be able to handle the pressure of a busy schedule, and you have to be able to not get discouraged if things don't always work out as planned. Inevitably there will be times when treatment won't work well, or patients won't be satisfied no matter what you do, so you have to be able to work with that. Having a pleasant disposition helps when dealing with patients, especially if they happen to be in pain and not in the best mood. A good disposition and a "we're all on the same team" approach works well with staff, too.

Q.   What are some of the pros and cons of your job?

A.   The pros of the job are extreme satisfaction when patients are thrilled about improved esthetics, or are out of intense pain due to something you've done for them. They are usually very, very appreciative. Your hours can be very flexible: you can work four long days and have three off, or work short days for six days, whatever suits you. You can work in any setting you'd like, a large, high-tech, group practice with specialists on site, or you can have a lower-key solo practice. You can specialize if a certain area interests you more, or have a general practice with more variety. Some of the cons are that although you work pretty much whatever hours you set, you do get emergencies at inopportune times. Usually you don't get many, but they are inevitable. In a larger practice this isn't as big a problem, as doctors cover for each other, but in a solo practice you're obligated to cover your emergencies whenever they occur. Sometimes money is an issue for patients, and you have to be able to compromise treatment to get the best result you can with what they can afford. There are patients even today with a tremendous fear of the dentist, so you have to be able to deal with people who are fearful, in pain, and not happy at all to see you.

Q.   What advice would you give to young people who are interested in the field?

A.   I would advise anyone interested in the field to visit a dental office and observe for a day, talk to the staff and especially the dentist, and get a feel for an average day. You might even want to work part-time in an office for a summer. If there is a dental school in your area, it might be good to visit that as well. I would also check out related fields if you're medically inclined, to see if any of them seem more appealing. It is also a good idea to evaluate your situation, your strengths and weaknesses. All medical fields require some strength in science, so if that isn't your interest, dentistry is probably not for you. You'll need a certain grade point average, especially in science, as admission is very competitive. A certain amount of manual dexterity is also very helpful in dentistry.

EMERGENCY MEDICAL TECHNICIANS

OVERVIEW

Emergency medical technicians (EMTs) are the first medical respondents at the scene of an accident, injury, crime, fire, or other emergency. They provide medical care to victims, including stopping bleeding, applying splints or braces to broken bones, or administering cardiopulmonary resuscitation, often while in transit to hospitals or medical facilities. EMTs also transfer patients between hospitals and other medical facilities for specialized treatment. Most work in ambulances, but some travel to accident scenes in special medically equipped helicopters. Duties of EMTs vary according to their level of training. Approximately 210,700 EMTs are employed in the United States. There will be good employment opportunities for EMTs through 2018.

FAST FACTS

High School Subjects
  Biology
  Health

Personal Skills
  Critical thinking
  Helping
  Judgment and decision making
  Technical

Minimum Education Level
  Some postsecondary training

Salary Range
  $19,000 to $30,000 to $51,000+

Employment Outlook
  About as fast as the average

O*NET-SOC
  29-2041.00

GOE
  04.04.01

DOT
  079

NOC
  3234

THE JOB

A horrible car-versus-semi crash. A four-alarm fire. A man suddenly collapses on a city street clutching his chest. Seconds after an emergency 911 call is placed, an emergency medical team is dispatched to provide help to victims in need. The work done by emergency medical technicians (EMTs) often means the difference between life and death. EMTs treat a wide spectrum of patients and their injuries including accidents, heart attacks, strokes, untimely birth deliveries, severe burns, and gunshot and stab wounds.

EMTs have different job titles based on their level of training. EMTs at the basic level (*EMT-Basic*) provide emergency assistance to assess, stabilize, and manage respiratory, cardiac, and trauma emergencies. They are trained to administer non-invasive emergency care. EMTs at the intermediate level (*EMT-Intermediate*) provide more advanced emergency care, including some invasive procedures, cardiac monitoring, intubations, and IVs. *Paramedics* have the highest level of training and are able to administer drug IVs, give defibrillation, and interpret electrocardiograms (EKGs). EMTs perform their duties under direct orders from doctors and nurses at a hospital or other health care facility.

EMTs are known for their quick thinking and immediate response to any situation, whether it is minor or critical. Dispatchers from a 911 center alert them to an emergency situation and its location. EMTs often arrive at the scene in a matter of minutes—usually in an ambulance, but sometimes in a helicopter or other mode of transportation. Once there, they determine the nature of the accident or illness. For example, if dispatched to a multi-car accident, EMTs determine the priority of injuries sustained. Sometimes, victims trapped in their vehicle must be freed before emergency care can be given. EMTs often work alongside police and firefighters to rescue victims, sometimes using rescue tools such as cutters, spreaders and rams that are frequently referred to as the "Jaws of Life." Once they have access to the victims, EMTs may ask victims to identify pain or discomfort if they are conscious; if not, EMTs take vital signs and visually assess the patient (including looking for medical alert bracelets or other identification to signal certain medical conditions).

Learn More About It

Cherry, Richard A. *SUCCESS! for the Paramedic.* 4th ed. Upper Saddle River, N.J.: Prentice Hall, 2007.

Clark, Joseph F. *My Ambulance Education: Life and Death on the Streets of the City.* Richmond Hill, O.N. Canada: Firefly Books, 2009.

Grayson, Steven. *A Paramedic's Story: Life, Death, and Everything in Between.* New York: Kaplan Publishing, 2010.

Ivey, Pat. *EMT: Beyond the Lights and Sirens.* New York: e-reads.com, 2009.

EMTs administer emergency care, depending on the condition of the victim and the extent of injuries sustained. They use bandages and gauze to control bleeding. They apply splints to set broken bones. A neck brace or backboard may be used if a neck or back injury is suspected. If the victim is short of breath, EMTs treat the individual with oxygen to help him or her regain a normal breathing pattern. If the victim is unconscious and does not appear to be breathing, EMTs administer CPR.

Once the victim is stabilized, EMTs use boards or stretchers to move him or her from the scene of the accident and into the ambulance for transportation. They make sure the victim is comfortable and securely strapped onto the stretcher. They monitor the victim en route to the hospital or other medical facility and administer medical care as needed. EMTs maintain communication with emergency department doctors and nurses regarding the condition of the patient. If the patient's condition or vital signs worsen during transport, doctors may advise EMT-Intermediates or paramedics to administer additional emergency care. EMT-Intermediates may start intravenous fluids or open airway passages by intubation. Paramedics may draw an IV line to administer drugs or use a defibrillator to shock a patient's stopped heart back into action. EMT-Intermediates and paramedics may also be asked by doctors to perform an EKG, interpret its results, and relay the information for review.

When the ambulance reaches the hospital, EMTs transfer the patient to the emergency room. They update doctors and nurses about the treatment they gave the patient at the scene and en-route.

EMTs also treat people suffering from injuries, accidents, or illness happening in their homes. For example, relatives of someone suffering from a heart attack or seriously injured from a fall may call 911 for emergency care. EMTs arrive at the scene and assess the situation. For a suspected heart attack, they take the patient's vital signs, including blood pressure and heart rate. EMTs may take an EKG reading or use bag-valve mask resuscitators for critical cases. They make sure the patient is stabilized before transferring him or her to the hospital.

After each run, EMTs clean and decontaminate their vehicle. This is especially important if they have treated patients with infectious diseases such as Hepatitis B and AIDS. They make sure instruments and equipment are maintained and medical supplies are replenished.

At the scene of a traffic accident, EMTs not traveling to the hospital with the victim may often help firefighters and police create a safe traffic environment. They light flares or use flashing signals to detour cars and pedestrians. If hazardous materials are present on the street, they use fire extinguishers or other equipment to absorb oil or harmful chemicals.

EMTs and paramedics also work with public agencies, schools, and community centers to educate the public about safety, or to teach first-aid programs.

EMTs usually work in teams of two or more; many times EMTs and paramedics work together as a pair, with the paramedic acting as team leader. A full-time EMT can expect to work 40 hours a week. Since accidents and illnesses occur 24 hours a day, EMTs work weekends and holidays.

EMTs work indoors and outdoors in all kinds of weather. This is an especially strenuous job. EMTs perform a considerable amount of kneeling, bending, and lifting. EMTs train to keep physically fit, yet despite this, they are often at risk for injuries. They are also at risk of catching communicable or infectious diseases, especially when dealing with high-risk patients such as those with AIDS or Hepatitis B.

EMTs face many stressful and traumatic situations. Patients sometimes die no matter how intense the efforts to save them. Others are injured so badly that they will have difficulty living productive lives. EMTs also risk injury when treating violent patients or those under the influence of drugs or alcohol. Most consider these challenges to be part of their job and enjoy helping people in need.

REQUIREMENTS

HIGH SCHOOL

You will need a high school diploma to enter an EMT training program. In high school, take classes in health, psychology, mathematics, biology, anatomy and physiology, and speech. Taking a foreign language such as Spanish will come in handy if you work in an area that has a large population that does not speak English as a first language.

POSTSECONDARY TRAINING

Training for EMTs is offered at several levels: EMT-Basic, EMT-Intermediate, and Paramedic. At the EMT-Basic level, students study the basics of emergency caregiving. They learn how to react to and manage medical emergencies such as respiratory distress, heart attacks, emergency childbirth, or broken bones, wounds, or other injuries caused by accidents, physical assaults, or other events. Their education includes both classroom time and experience out in the field with experienced EMTs. Training requirements for those at the EMT-Intermediate level vary by state. According to the U.S. Department of Labor, "EMTs at the nationally defined levels, EMT-Intermediate 1985 and EMT-Intermediate 1999, typically require 30 to 350 hours of training based on scope of practice. Students learn advanced skills such the use of advanced airway devices, intravenous fluids, and some medications." Paramedics receive the most advanced training, which often culminates in the awarding of an associate's or bachelor's degree. The Commission on Accreditation of Allied Health Education Programs accredits paramedic education programs. Visit its website, www.caahep.org/Find-An-Accredited-Program, for a list of accredited programs.

CERTIFICATION AND LICENSING

The National Registry of Emergency Medical Technicians offers certification to emergency medical service providers at five levels: first responder (a designation that is typically held by police officers and firefighters); EMT-Basic; EMT-Intermediate (which has two levels called 1985 and 1999), and paramedic. Additionally, some states have their own certification programs.

All 50 states and the District of Columbia require EMTs to be licensed. Licensing requirements vary by state. Some states have their own licensing examinations and also require EMTs to be certified by the National Registry of Emergency Medical Technicians.

OTHER REQUIREMENTS

To be a successful EMT, you should be calm under pressure, decisive, and emotionally stable, since you will occasionally encounter heartbreaking or stressful situations. Other important traits include good overall physical condition (including dexterity, good eyesight and accurate color vision, and endurance to lift heavy loads), the ability to work as a member of a team, and strong communication skills.

EXPLORING

There are many ways to learn more about a career as an EMT. You can read books and magazines about the field, take first-aid and CPR classes offered by the Red Cross or other organizations, and visit the websites of college EMT programs to learn about typical classes and possible career paths, and ask your teacher or school counselor to arrange an information interview with an EMT.

EMPLOYERS

Approximately 210,700 EMTs are employed in the United States. EMTs work for private ambulance companies, fire departments, police departments, public emergency service agencies, and hospitals. While the majority of EMTs work in paid positions in urban areas, some work in volunteer positions in small, rural communities.

GETTING A JOB

Many EMTs obtain their first jobs as a result of contacts made through college internships, career fairs, or networking events. Others seek assistance in obtaining job leads from college career services offices, newspaper want ads, and employment websites.

ADVANCEMENT

EMTs advance by receiving higher pay and by gaining additional training to move from EMT-Basic, to EMT-Intermediate, to paramedic. Paramedics can also advance to supervisory positions. With additional training, some EMTs become teachers, dispatchers, physician assistants, registered nurses, physicians, or sales or marketing professionals for emergency medical equipment manufacturers.

EARNINGS

Salaries for emergency medical technicians vary by type of employer, geographic region, and the worker's experience, education, and skill level. Median annual salaries for EMTs were $30,000 in 2009, according to the U.S. Department of Labor (USDL). Salaries ranged from less than $19,360 to $51,460 or more. The USDL reports the following mean annual earnings for EMTs by employer: state government, $49,560; local government, $36,780; general medical and surgical hospitals, $33,390; and other ambulatory health care services, $30,110.

Emergency medical technicians usually receive benefits such as health and life insurance, vacation days, sick leave, and a savings and pension plan. Part-time workers must provide their own benefits.

EMPLOYMENT OUTLOOK

Employment for EMTs is expected to grow about as fast as the average for all careers through 2018, according to the U.S. Department of Labor

(USDL). Growth is occurring as a result of an increase in the U.S. population—especially among the elderly, who typically require more medical care than other age groups. Opportunities will be especially good in cities and with private ambulance services. The USDL reports that "competition will be greater for jobs in local government, including fire, police, and independent third-service rescue squad departments that tend to have better salaries and benefits." EMTs who receive advanced certifications and education will have the best job prospects.

FOR MORE INFORMATION

For industry information, contact
American Ambulance Association
8400 Westpark Drive, Second Floor
McLean, VA 22102-5116
www.the-aaa.org

For career information, contact
**National Association of
Emergency Medical Technicians**
PO Box 1400
Clinton, MS 39060-1400
info@naemt.org
www.naemt.org

For information on certification, contact
**National Registry of
Emergency Medical Technicians**
Rocco V. Morando Building
6610 Busch Boulevard
PO Box 29233
Columbus, OH 43229-1740
www.nremt.org

Interview: Jerry Johnston

Jerry Johnston is an emergency medical technician and the past president of the National Association of Emergency Medical Technicians. He discussed his career with the editors of *Hot Health Care Careers*.

Q. What made you want to enter this career?

A. My father owned an ambulance service. So, while most kids were flipping burgers and delivering newspapers, I was working with my dad. When I turned 16, he allowed me to go on interfacility transfers. (You'll have to remember, this was the early to middle 70's; there were no EMS laws yet.) EMT training had just begun and was thought of as the gold standard then. About that time, the TV show "Emergency" came onto the air. That sealed the deal for me. All I ever wanted to do was work as a paramedic. I was fortunate enough to attend college and complete my degree in business. I knew someday I wanted to lead an EMS organization, and I thought that degree, combined with my EMS background and experience, would prepare me well.

Q. What is one thing that young people may not know about a career as an EMT?

A. It can be equally rewarding as well as frustrating. You might deliver a baby one day, and watch someone die the next, knowing that you did everything in your power to save them...but it just wasn't to be.

Q. **What are the most important personal and professional qualities for EMTs?**

A. Commitment and dedication, and a realization that this career is one of lifelong learning. Medicine is an ever-changing science, and you must be dedicated to being a lifetime learner. This is not a profession that once you are finished with your initial training you are done... actually, you have just begun.

Q. **What are some of the pros and cons of being an EMT?**

A. Pros: No two days are ever alike. You may run calls like crazy one day and sit the next. Because of that, you need to be in a constant state of readiness. You are privileged to take care of people when they are having a particularly bad day. That is an awesome responsibility, but one, when taken seriously, that provides you with the opportunity to make a significant impact in that person's life.

Cons: We're never closed. This is a 24/7/365 business. Because of that, someone always has to work the night shift, holidays, maybe your child's birthday... it's just part of the job. You accept that when you are in training. It also can be dangerous, from driving and working in the emergency vehicle to working in austere environments. You need a good sense of situational awareness.

Q. **What advice would you give to young people who are interested in becoming EMTs?**

A. Pay particular attention to your study of math and sciences. That will make your training much easier. Do your homework—that is, prepare yourself for what is expected. Visit your local EMS organization. Ask questions; do ride-alongs (if permitted). Try to gain as much of an understanding about all the aspects of the job as you can before you spend your time and money on the education.

Q. **Can you tell us about the National Association of Emergency Medical Technicians (NAEMT)? How important is association membership to career success?**

A. NAEMT is the only national association for all EMS professionals, representing the interests of more than 30,000 members. Professional associations make a difference. I have seen firsthand their positive effects and influence. I believe it is incumbent on any professional to not only belong to his or her professional association, but to be engaged. Professional associations can be very influential with good leadership and an engaged membership. In NAEMT, members have the opportunity to have a voice on Capitol Hill and beyond, and to be involved in committee work and educational programs, and even run for office, all for the betterment of EMS.

HEALTH AIDES

OVERVIEW

Health aides help patients who are elderly, sick, or physically or mentally disabled with their daily living activities. These activities are conducted in the patients' homes, though aides often accompany patients to medical appointments and other activities. Some aides are certified to provide medical assessment or help with therapy exercises. Health aides learn their skills via on-the-job training. About 1.7 million health aides are employed in the United States. Employment for health aides is expected to be excellent.

THE JOB

Many people who are ill, injured, or infirm want to stay in their own homes instead of living in a residential, long-

FAST FACTS

High School Subjects
Family and consumer science
Health
Personal Skills
Communication
Following instructions
Helping
Minimum Education Level
High school diploma
Salary Range
$15,000 to $20,000 to $29,000+
Employment Outlook
Much faster than the average
O*NET-SOC
31-1011.00, 39-9021.00
GOE
14.07.01
DOT
354
NOC
3413

term care facility or nursing home. However, they require a degree of care that their family or friends are incapable of providing. In these cases, many people turn to the services of *home health aides* or *personal care aides* (also known as *homemakers, caregivers, companions,* and *personal attendants)* for assistance.

Home health aides and personal-care aides share many of the same duties, with some differences, especially in regards to their employer. Home health aides work for certified home health agencies or hospice agencies. These agencies receive government funding, and so they must comply with state regulations. Personal-care aides work for public or private agencies supplying health care services.

Home health aides travel from site to site, providing skilled care to people of all ages. They complete medical and/or psychological assessments, maintain records, and note any changes in their client's condition. They work alongside other health care professionals such as nurses or therapists. Their duties include cleaning and dressing wounds, administering medications, and educating patients and their families about patients' particular diseases or conditions. Some home health aides are trained to assist patients with daily physical, speech, or occupational therapy exercises as prescribed by health care professionals.

Some home health aides also provide non-medical care to patients, as do personal and home care aides. Their duties include helping patients with the many activities of daily living. Aides help patients take baths and showers, or perform daily grooming, such as brushing patients' teeth or combing their hair. They also help patients get dressed or undressed. Other daily responsibilities include bringing patients to the toilet throughout the day, transferring them in and out of wheelchairs, and assisting them in walking or climbing and descending stairs. Aides also help patients during mealtimes by preparing their food and helping them eat, if needed. They make sure that patients eat to maintain their strength, as well as take their medications at the appropriate times.

Depending on the time spent with a patient, aides may do light housework, laundry, or other tasks around the house. At times, they may accompany patients to the grocery store, the doctor's office, or on another appointments or errands. Patients sometimes ask their aides to help them use the telephone or even manage their finances.

Aside from the many tasks done by home health aides and home care aides, equally important is the sense of psychological support and well-being they give to their patients. Patients, as well their concerned families, feel comforted knowing a reliable person is available to help with daily tasks and provide companionship.

Most aides work full time, about 40 hours a week. They often work evenings or weekends to accommodate patients' needs. The work is demanding, both physically and emotionally.

Some tasks done by health aides are unpleasant—emptying bedpans or Foley catheter bags, changing soiled bed linens or clothing, or cleaning patients when they become incontinent. Patients can sometimes become irritable, stubborn, angry, or disoriented and can be quite difficult to handle. Regardless of the challenges they face, health aides perform their duties with compassion for their patients.

Oftentimes, health aides care for multiple patients—up to five a day—working with each for a few hours before moving on to the next client. Health aides should be able to shift gears easily, adapting for a variety of patient personalities, situations, and work environments.

Most aides work independently, with occasional visits from health professionals, their supervisor, or manager. They must have a reliable vehicle, or access to another mode of transportation, in order to travel from patient to patient.

REQUIREMENTS

HIGH SCHOOL

Take health, psychology, and family and consumer science courses in high school. Since you will need strong communication skills to interact effectively with your clients and coworkers, it is a good idea to take as many speech and English classes as possible. Taking a foreign language such as Spanish will come in handy if you work in an area that has a large population that does not speak English as a first language.

POSTSECONDARY TRAINING

Health aides typically do not need to have a high school diploma, but it is always a good idea to graduate from high school since you will need at least a high school education, and at least some college training, to work in most careers. Aides learn their skills via on-the-job training from licensed practical nurses, registered nurses, experienced aides, and managers. They learn how to cook and clean, feed patients, recognize health issues, and react effectively during emergencies.

CERTIFICATION AND LICENSING

Health aides can receive national certification from the National Association for Home Care and Hospice (NAHC). Certification, while voluntary, is highly recommended. It is an excellent way to stand out from other job applicants and demonstrate your abilities to prospective employers.

Health aides who are employed by agencies that receive reimbursement from Medicaid or Medicare must complete a minimum 75-hour training program and a competency evaluation or state certification program. Many employers require aides to complete the NAHC's certification program as proof of competency. Requirements vary by state. Contact your state's department of licensing for more information on requirements in your state.

OTHER REQUIREMENTS

Health aides must be in excellent physical condition. They frequently move patients in and out of beds or wheelchairs, or support them as they descend stairs, cross streets, or get in and out of vehicles. Aides should be strong and physically fit, especially when working with obese patients or those with limited mobility. Since lift apparatus are not often found in patient's homes, aides must lift and shift patients, following procedures to prevent injury to themselves. Other important traits for health aides include compassion for people who are suffering from illness, injury, or old age; excellent communication skills; patience; an upbeat personality; and strong ethics, since you will be working in patients' homes and trusted with their well-being.

EXPLORING

There are many ways to learn more about a career as a health aide. You can read books and magazines (such as *Caring*, http://digitalcaring magazine.nahc.org) about the field. You can ask your health teacher or school counselor to arrange an information interview with a health aide. If you are in high school, you could try to land a job as a health aide with a home health care service or at a nursing home. This will give you a chance to see if the duties of a health aide are a good fit for your interests and abilities.

EMPLOYERS

Approximately 1.7 million health aides are employed in the United States. Most work for home health care services, residential care facilities, individual and family services, and private households. A few operate their own businesses.

GETTING A JOB

Many health aides obtain job leads from newspaper want ads and employment websites. Additionally, national- and state-level professional associations, such as the National Association for Home Care and Hospice (NAHCH), provide job listings at their websites. The NAHCH career website can be found at www.homecarecareers.com.

ADVANCEMENT

Other than salary increases, health aides have few ways of advancing unless they continue their education. Those who go back to school can become nursing aides, licensed practical nurses, registered nurses, or health care managers. Self-employed aides may start their own businesses.

EARNINGS

Salaries for home health aides vary by type of employer, geographic region, and the worker's experience, education, and skill level. Median annual salaries for home health aides were $20,480 in 2009, according to the U.S. Department of Labor. Salaries ranged from less than $15,950 to $29,390 or more. Salaries for personal and home care aides ranged from less than $15,300 to $25,890 or more, with a median of $19,680.

Health aides usually receive benefits such as health and life insurance, vacation days, sick leave, and a savings and pension plan. Self-employed workers must provide their own benefits.

EMPLOYMENT OUTLOOK

Employment for health aides is expected to grow much faster than the average for all careers through 2018, according to the U.S. Department of Labor. In fact, the careers of home health aide and personal-care aide are expected to grow by 46 percent through 2018—adding 836,700 new jobs during this time span. Several factors are fueling growth. The U.S. population is continuing to grow, and the number of people—especially elderly people—needing care is increasing rapidly. Health care costs in hospitals and other nonresidential settings are rising, which is prompting more people to seek care in their own homes. There is also high turnover in this career because the pay is low and work responsibilities are demanding. Many young people view this career as a stepping-stone to other health care careers in nursing, therapy, or health care management.

FOR MORE INFORMATION

For information on certification and statistics about home health care, visit the following Web site.
National Association for Home Care and Hospice
228 Seventh Street, SE
Washington, DC 20003-4306
202-547-7424
www.nahc.org

HEALTH CARE MANAGERS AND ADMINISTRATORS

OVERVIEW

Health care managers and administrators, also known as *health care executives* and *medical and health services managers,* plan, direct, coordinate, and supervise the delivery of health care services. They work at hospitals, clinics, nursing homes, home health agencies, private offices, and other health care facilities. A master's degree in health care management or a related field is required for employment at large facilities; a bachelor's degree may be sufficient for entry-level positions at small facilities. Approximately 283,500 medical and health services managers are employed in the United States. Employment is expected to be good through 2018.

FAST FACTS

High School Subjects
Business
Mathematics
Personal Skills
Communication
Leadership
Organizational
Time management
Minimum Education Level
Bachelor's degree
Salary Range
$44,000 to $81,000 to $140,000+
Employment Outlook
Faster than the average
O*NET-SOC
11-9111.00
GOE
14.01.01
DOT
187
NOC
0014

THE JOB

Health care managers and administrators are responsible for the operations of a health care facility, including its clinical health services, financial office, human resources department, educational programs (some facilities offer training to health care students), security, janitorial services, information technology department, and other departments.

A large part of a manager's job involves managing the daily fiscal operations of the facility. Managers look for ways to reduce costs without sacrificing quality health care for patients. This entails keeping up to date on insurance policies, changes in Medicare or Medicaid reimbursements, and federal laws or regulations regarding health care reform.

Health care managers oversee improvements to equipment and medical technology, building repairs and additions, and the procurement of medications, equipment, and supplies. At least once a year, state health inspectors visit the facility to make sure it meets health regulations. Violations may result in fines or, in severe cases, a forced shut-down. Health care managers ensure their facilities are safe and up to standards as mandated by the state.

Supervision of personnel is another duty. Health care managers often interview potential employees and have final say in employee hiring and firing. They are in charge of training and continuing education offered to staff members. They establish pay scales and sometimes are asked for input regarding benefits packages offered to staff members. Health care managers also mediate disputes between employees or address complaints made by patients or family members.

Security is another important duty. Health care managers ensure that employees and patients at their facilities are physically safe while on the hospital's premises. Health care managers also ensure patient privacy and confidentiality by protecting the security of all patient records, whether in paper or electronic format. Recent government regulations mandate that all health care facilities and providers maintain patient records in secure electronic format. Health care managers, as well as select staff and department members, must participate in service training to keep up to date on changing computer and software technology.

Health care managers meet regularly with department heads, such as the director of nursing or the medical director. These meetings provide department heads with an opportunity to update the administrator regarding current or future projects and to air any grievances.

Health care managers often act as their facilities' representative for community functions and events. They participate in community outreach programs and health fairs that educate the public on health issues.

Duties and responsibilities of health care managers vary by facility. Large facilities such as hospitals may have several assistant administrators who manage clinical departments such as therapy, nursing, surgery, and medical records and health information. For example, the nursing department is managed by the director of nursing, and the medical records department or therapy departments are supervised by separate managers. These managers typically have experience in their department's specialty. For example, a director of physical therapy is typically a practicing physical therapist. A director of nursing typically is a nurse with advanced education. There are managers who supervise security, information technology, janitorial services, billing, and other departments. All departmental managers report to the head hospital administrator. At facilities that are smaller in size, such as a nursing home, administrators may handle all daily activities as well as issues regarding personnel, faculty operations, admissions, and resident care. Some medical practices employ medical administrators to manage the business aspect of the practice, including staff, billing, budgeting, equipment procurement, and overall patient flow.

Full-time health care managers work five days a week for about 40 hours a week. However, since many health care facilities operate 24 hours a day, health care managers and administrators often work long hours, including those at night and on weekends, to manage any crisis or emergency situations that arise. They carry pagers or dedicated cell phones for

Debunking Common Misconceptions About Health Care Careers

Health care is the largest industry in the United States, according to the U.S. Department of Labor. It employs 14.3 million people, features 12 of the top 20 fastest-growing occupations, and offers great opportunities to those with less than a four-year college education, as well as those, such as physicians and advanced practice nurses, with advanced education. And the industry continues to grow: about 19 percent (or 3.6 million) of all new jobs created between 2004 and 2014 will be in health care.

Despite this rapid growth and the large number of people employed in the field, many people have misconceptions about the health care industry that keep them from reaching their career potential. Here are a few of the most common health care career myths and the facts about them.

Myth #1: All health care professionals work in hospitals and medical centers.
The Facts. Employment in these settings was the norm for years, but, today, health care professionals—especially registered nurses, physicians, and thera- pists—work in a variety of nontraditional settings. These include staffing or recruitment agencies, managed care companies, professional associations, insurance companies, publishing companies, occupational health companies, research facilities, law firms, private corporations, and colleges and universities.

Myth #2: The nursing shortage means that you will get any job that you want.
The Facts. Yes, you will definitely get a job at some point, but your job search may take longer than you expect—especially if you have not received specialized training. Additionally, some hospitals do not hire new graduates to work in demanding specialties such as critical care nursing.

Myth #3: Medical technician, nursing, and other health care positions require a four-year degree.
The Facts. Not true for many careers. Many employers—especially due to the nursing shortage—are hiring nurses with two-year associate degrees from community colleges. Other rewarding careers that only require an associate degree include occupational therapy assistant, physical therapist assistant, respiratory therapist, and radiologic technologist.

such emergencies. Health care managers and administrators work in com- fortable, well-lit offices.

Many health care managers have limited patient contact, instead spend- ing much of their time dealing with policy issues or other changes needed to make their institutions or departments run smoothly. This in turn serves the patient population. They deal with insurance companies, Medicare or Medicaid, government health service agencies, medical contractors, and medical supply companies to ensure the efficient operation of their facilities.

Health care managers and administrators supervise the work of assistant administrators or managers. Some travel may be necessary to attend meetings and community events, or to inspect satellite facilities.

REQUIREMENTS

HIGH SCHOOL

High school classes that will be useful for aspiring health care managers include business, computer science, health, mathematics, English, and speech.

POSTSECONDARY TRAINING

A master's degree is required for employment at large health care facilities; a bachelor's degree may be sufficient for entry-level positions at small facilities. Most people earn a graduate degree in health services administration, long-term care administration, health sciences, or public health. Others pursue graduate degrees in business or public administration, with a concentration in health care management, or seek joint degrees in business administration and public health. The Commission on Accreditation of Healthcare Management Education (www.cahme.org) accredits graduate-level health care management programs. The Association of University Programs in Health Administration offers a list of baccalaureate, master's, and doctoral health care management programs at its website, www.aupha.org. Offices of physicians and other health care facilities sometimes hire managers with extensive on-the-job experience but no college degree.

CERTIFICATION AND LICENSING

Voluntary certification is offered by several professional associations including the American Health Information Management Association, the American College of Health Care Administrators, the American Medical Directors Association, the Professional Association of Health Care Office Management, and the American College of Medical Practice Executives. Certification, while voluntary, is highly recommended. It is an excellent way to stand out from other job applicants and demonstrate your abilities to prospective employers.

The U.S. Department of Labor reports that "all states and the District of Columbia require nursing care facility administrators to have a bachelor's degree, pass a licensing examination, complete a state-approved training program, and pursue continuing education. Some states also require licenses for administrators in assisted-living facilities. A license is not required in other areas of medical and health services management." The National Association of Long Term Care Administrator Boards offers information on state licensing at its website, www.nabweb.org.

OTHER REQUIREMENTS

Health care managers must have strong leadership abilities to effectively lead staff members and inspire them to provide excellent health care services to patients. They should be decisive, organized, diplomatic, flexible, and good at solving problems. Strong communication skills are important because they frequently interact with other managers, staff members, inspectors, and others. Health care managers must have excellent financial management skills and strong ethics, since they are tasked with managing multimillion dollar budgets and making financial decisions that will affect the future of the facility and the quality of the health care services provided to patients.

EXPLORING

There are many ways to learn more about a career as a health care manager. You can read books [such as *Opportunities in Hospital Administration Careers*, by I. Donald Snook (McGraw-Hill, 2006)] and journals about the field, visit the websites of college health care management programs to learn about typical classes and possible career paths, and ask your teacher or school counselor to arrange an information interview with a health care manager. Professional associations can also provide information about the field. The American College of Healthcare Executives provide a wealth of information on health care managers and careers at its website, Make a Difference: Discover a Career in Healthcare Management! (www. healthmanagementcareers.org). You should also try to land a part-time job in a medical office. This will give you a chance to interact with health care managers and see if the career is a good fit for your interests and abilities.

EMPLOYERS

Approximately 283,500 medical and health services managers are employed in the United States. Medical and health services managers are employed by hospitals; HMOs; centers for cardiac rehabilitation, urgent care, and diagnostic imaging; group medical practices; offices of health practitioners; nursing homes; adult day care programs; home health care agencies; and other residential facilities.

GETTING A JOB

Many health care managers obtain their first jobs as a result of contacts made through college internships, career fairs, or networking events. Others seek assistance in obtaining job leads from college career services offices, newspaper want ads, and employment websites. Additionally, professional associations, such as the American College of Health Care Administrators and the American College of Healthcare Executives, provide job listings at their websites. See For More Information for contact information. Those interested in positions with the federal government should visit the U.S. Office of Personnel Management's website, www.usajobs.opm.gov.

ADVANCEMENT

Health care managers advance by receiving increases in pay or promotions to higher positions, by moving to larger facilities, and by working as consultants or college professors.

EARNINGS

Salaries for health care managers vary by type of employer, geographic region, and the worker's experience, education, and skill level. Median annual salaries for health care managers were $81,850 in 2009, according to the U.S. Department of Labor (USDL). Salaries ranged from less than $49,750 to $140,300 or more. The USDL reports the following mean annual earnings for health care managers by employer: general medical and surgical hospitals, $96,660; offices of physicians, $88,650; outpatient care centers, $84,980; home health care services, $83,160; and nursing care facilities, $77,560.

Office managers in specialty physicians' practices earned the following average total compensation in 2009, according to the Professional Association of Health Care Office Management: cardiology, $58,899; gastroenterology, $54,314; dermatology, $54,201; pediatrics, $51,466; orthopedics, $51,263; internal medicine, $48,814; ophthalmology, $48,793; family practice, $47,152; and obstetrics and gynecology, $44,910.

Employers offer a variety of benefits, including the following: medical, dental, and life insurance; paid holidays, vacations, and sick and personal days; 401(k) plans; profit-sharing plans; retirement and pension plans; and educational-assistance programs. Health care managers who work as freelance consultants must provide their own benefits.

Other Career Options in Health Care

- ✔ Biomedical Equipment Technicians
- ✔ Chiropractors
- ✔ Dental Laboratory Technicians
- ✔ Dietitians and Nutritionists
- ✔ Clinical Laboratory Technologists and Technicians
- ✔ Health Advocates
- ✔ Histologic Technicians
- ✔ Holistic Physicians
- ✔ Kinesiologists
- ✔ Medical Ethicists
- ✔ Nursing Home Administrators
- ✔ Ophthalmologists
- ✔ Optometrists
- ✔ Orthotists and Prosthetists
- ✔ Perfusionists
- ✔ Respiratory Therapists and Technicians
- ✔ Transplant Coordinators

EMPLOYMENT OUTLOOK

The U.S. Department of Labor predicts that employment for health care managers will grow faster than the average for all careers through 2018. Opportunities will be best in offices of health practitioners, general medical and surgical hospitals, home health care services, and outpatient care centers. There will also be increasing opportunities at health care management companies that provide management services to health care facilities on a contract basis. Health care managers who oversee care for the elderly (from independent assisted-living facilities to supervised 24-hour care) will have especially strong job prospects.

FOR MORE INFORMATION

For information on certification and state licensing, contact
American College of Health Care Administrators
1321 Duke Street, Suite 400
Alexandria, VA 22314-3563
202-536-5120
www.achca.org

For information on education, careers, and certification, contact
American College of Healthcare Executives
One North Franklin Street, Suite 1700
Chicago, IL 60606-3529
312-424-2800
geninfo@ache.org
www.ache.org

Contact the association for information about medical directors who work in long-term care.
American Medical Directors Association
11000 Broken Land Parkway, Suite 400
Columbia, MD 21044-3532
800-876-2632
www.amda.com

For information on accredited programs and careers, contact
Association of University Programs in Health Administration
2000 North 14th Street, Suite 780
Arlington, VA 22201-2543
703-894-0940
aupha@aupha.org
www.aupha.org

For information on certification, contact
Medical Group Management Association
104 Inverness Terrace East
Englewood, CO 80112-5306
877-275-6462
www.mgma.org

To learn more about careers in health care office management and certification, contact
Professional Association of Health Care Office Management
1576 Bella Cruz Drive, Suite 360
Lady Lake, FL 32159-8969
800-451-9311
www.pahcom.com

Interview: Joan Rissmiller

Joan Rissmiller, CMM is a medical practice administrator at Bausch and Jones Eye Associates in Allentown, Pennsylvania. She has worked in the field for 26 years. Joan discussed her career with the editors of *Hot Health Care Careers*.

Q. What made you want to enter this career?

**A. ** I always considered the field of medicine to be fascinating. The thought of working with physicians and patients seeking medical advice and care was the inspiring factor. I started working part-time in a local hospital and had the opportunity to work in many areas of the hospital including the emergency room. From the first day I stepped into the hospital, I knew that health care was the career for me. I am a people person, and I wanted to make a difference in patients' lives.

Q. If you could do anything different in preparing for your career in college/high school, what would it be?

A. Education, education, education. Privately owned practices are becoming extinct. They are being sold to hospitals and management corporations. In order to succeed in this business environment, you need to have at least a B.S. degree but preferably an MBA in health care management in order to acquire positions at the top of the corporate structure.

Q. What are some of the pros and cons of your job?

A. It is a rewarding career. When your act of kindness and concern puts a smile on the face of a patient who is battling a terminal illness, suddenly your paycheck is immaterial. When you fight a battle with an insurance company and come out the victor, what a sense of triumph and accomplishment. When you manage a large staff and at least half of them adore their job and love coming to work, you realize that you do make a difference. Working with physicians who are dedicated to their profession and their patients makes you appreciate the magnitude of providing exceptional health care to those in need. What an adrenaline rush when you realize that you play a part in the health care needs of so many individuals and that your presence has a tremendous effect on so many lives.

It is a turbulent profession governed by federal, state, and insurance guiding principles. It is very difficult to keep abreast of the constant changes and updated adherence policies. It is challenging to budget and plan for the future of your practice when there are so many unexpected outside influences.

Q. What advice would you give to young people who are interested in the field? What are the best ways to find a job?

A. Be patient. It takes a lot of time and many years of experience to make it to the top. Take the time to learn the various positions in the practice. It will provide you with a sense and appreciation of the tasks that your staff has to handle, and your staff will respect you for taking an interest in their role in the practice. Join professional organizations that will offer the opportunity to network and attend annual conferences. You need to get out there and stay connected.

Throughout my years, I found the best way to obtain the better employment opportunities is through word of mouth from other practice managers or professional acquaintances. That being said, again I emphasize the significance of joining professional organizations and networking.

I have come to realize that there are a lot of jobs that are not advertised in the local newspapers, since the Internet is now a great tool to obtain employment opportunities. Check the employment opportunity listings at local hospitals.

In closing, [the newspaper publisher] Katharine Graham's quotation explicitly relates my passion for my practice management job: "To love what you do and feel that it matters, how could anything be more fun?"

Interview: Janet Burch

Janet Burch, CMM is the administrator at Pikes Peak Nephrology Associates PC, in Colorado Springs, Colorado. She was the Professional Association of Health Care Office Management Medical Manager of the Year in 2009. Janet discussed her career with the editors of *Hot Health Care Careers*.

Q. What made you want to enter this career?

A. My career in health care management has been a fortunate series of unplanned events, and not at all by design. In fact, I didn't enter health care with any expectation of starting a career——I simply needed a job.

An employment counselor sent me on a job assignment to work in the medical records room of a five-physician practice. I had a high school diploma and little work experience. Since I entered the practice in an entry-level position, the only direction I could go was up (or out!).

By keeping my eyes and ears open, and modeling my behaviors after the more successful employees in the practice, it wasn't long before I was given opportunities to learn new skills. With new skills, doors opened. Within a few years, I was doing work I wouldn't have imagined I could do in those early days in the medical records room.

Inspired, I pursued higher education, earning a B.S. in business management and a M.B.A. in health care management. Together, years of experience combined with a formal education helped give me confidence that my employment in health care management was more than just a job. To maintain that edge, my affiliations with professional associations add polish to my skill sets and keep the work I perform relevant to my own personal and professional goals. The work has become the reward that feeds my desire to continue in this field.

Q. What is one thing that young people may not know about a career as a health care manager?

A. Health care managers in small medical practices are health care's ultimate generalists. Their job requires them to be experts in nearly everything. They are the people everyone in the organization turns to with questions and problems. Next to the physician, they are often the organization's most important resource.

To illustrate, health care managers are the organization's compliance officers and risk managers. They must understand the legal and regulatory environment governing health care activities. They are also financial officers. The role requires health care managers to analyze the financial status of the accounts receivable and accounts payable, and to negotiate and manage the terms of multiple managed-care agreements. Their role is to make the organization profitable and efficient, and to minimize expenses. Not only must health care managers know these critical elements, they must be able to discuss their analyses with multiple stakeholders.

Health care managers support all of the organization's HR management functions, from recruiting to termination and everything that occurs in between. Not only must they be familiar with employment law, health care managers must also establish and enforce policies to provide a safe working environment. Health care managers must possess a working knowledge of a third-party reimbursement system that includes medical documentation, billing, and coding. They must understand departmental workflows to help overcome obstacles that impede the organization's overall efficiency. In a competitive environment, marketing and public relations are necessary skills for health care managers. They are often the front-line support for technical glitches and equipment malfunctions.

The use of electronic health records (EHR) opens new opportunities to use technical and analytical skills. Data that was once buried within the pages of paper records is more easily extracted once an EHR system becomes functional. Consider product recall information and the daunting task of identifying the records of a handful of patients who might have received recalled pharmaceutical samples out of thousands of paper records. With greater access to and more data available, quality reporting and disease management become increasingly important data elements for health care managers to understand as reimbursement shifts from fee-for-service to outcomes measurement.

Health care managers must also possess exceptional people and communication skills, as relationships in this line of work are critically important. These skills are the essence of a health care manager's role. The success of every action performed by a health care manager depends heavily upon the actions of others. Decisions are made upon the information available, and the better the sources of your information, the better your decisions will be. Treat the people around you with respect. Trust and verify. Additionally, resourcefulness, maximum flexibility, and a sense of humor are absolute requirements in this position.

Q.   What are your primary and secondary job duties?

A.   Like any other management position, my duties are best summarized as leading, planning, organizing, and controlling. My role is to help the physicians fulfill the organization's mission and to do so in a manner that adds value to the lives of everyone it touches.

Variety is not lacking. Some days are spent lobbying legislators on health care issues important to physicians. Other days are spent behind the desk reviewing our stats, crunching numbers, and analyzing opportunities. I often observe activities within the organization and speak with staff members. It is important to look for actions that are done well, and ones that can be improved.

Weekly meetings with the physicians help keep everyone informed. Members of our management team and I also meet monthly, and more often as needed. I am active in the community meeting with other health care providers to market our services and arrange educational outreach. With rapid changes occurring in health care administration, reading and research occupy a good many hours of my time.

Communicating this information to the physicians and staff is an ongoing responsibility. Similarly, the exchange of information from physicians and staff to me often sets the stage for work to be accomplished to improve patient care, improve profitability, or, in some other manner, improve the activities of the organization.

Q.   What are the most important qualities for people in your career?

A.   The attributes that appear in the most successful people in health care management are ones that are present in other professional services.

Integrity, honesty, and a strong desire to perform meaningful work are qualities that will serve an individual well in this field.

A successful health care manager must be flexible and resilient, as pressure to change the health care delivery system is having a profound effect on the manner in which our work is performed. Every day, it seems, brings new information about changes that will affect the organization next week, next month, next year, and beyond.

Success also means working as part of a team and drawing upon the group's strengths. Developing and maintaining healthy work relationships is important, since everyone's contribution to patient care and the profitability of the organization counts. An interest in promoting one's individual agenda probably won't work well in these situations.

Success also means that we can never be satisfied that good is good enough. Our actions are public. It's important to give our best at all times, give credit where it's due, and acknowledge when we can't meet expectations.

Q.   What advice would you give to young people who are interested in the field? What are the best ways to find a job?

A.   Unlike my experience, young people will be better poised for a career in health care management with the benefit of a formal education. Experience will come, but education is the best pathway to understanding what is required of a health care manager. Health care management, as it is today, is an unwieldy, nonconforming beast. It is complex, highly regulated, convoluted in nature, but not impossible to learn if you would like to work in a challenging and rewarding career. The next few years promise rapid, sweeping changes. Any edge you can gain through your efforts will make the job much more manageable.

Add an internship or mentoring experience to your learning experience, and the combination of classroom and "real life" skills should help launch a successful career. Work with your school counselor, or seek a mentor on your own who can help you break into the field. Volunteering is also an excellent way to observe and meet people in health care who can help you decide if the career path is the right one for you.

Q.   What has been one (or more) of the most rewarding experiences in your career and why?

A.   When you can contribute to the success of something bigger than you are, you are left with a sense of fulfillment. Sometimes it is as simple as seeing a patient smile and forget his or her problems for a brief moment. Often it is stepping back, listening to others, and seeing resolution to a lingering problem from a different perspective. These actions offer a sense of satisfaction.

Perhaps the experiences that mean the most in the course of a career are those that are a result of relationships. Health care is a service industry, and a number of those who serve seem to have truly remarkable talents. It is doubly rewarding to have relationships with the providers of health care and the people who support them, and to be a part of their efforts to improve the lives of the people in our community.

HEALTH INFORMATION MANAGEMENT SPECIALISTS

OVERVIEW

Health information management specialists, also known as *health information management technicians,* capture, analyze, and protect patients' medical information. This information is stored in paper or electronic format. Information they coordinate includes patients' medical history, diagnoses, laboratory tests, x-ray and other diagnostic procedure reports, and treatment plans. An associate's degree is typically required to enter the field. Approximately 277,700 medical records and health information management technicians are employed in the United States. Employment opportunities are expected to be very good through 2018.

THE JOB

Every time a patient goes to the emergency room, is admitted to the hospital, visits a primary care physician for an annual physical, or undergoes laboratory tests, a record is made of that visit or procedure, as well as every referral or second-opinion consultation. The notes taken during an actual examination or procedure are considered the "primary patient record." It includes patient data, which physicians use to get a better idea of a patient's medical condition. Primary patient records also include any documentation, observations, or instructions made by the physician. A "secondary patient record" is created from information taken from the primary record and includes data pertinent to nonclinical people such as administration, regulation, and billing/payment history. The collection of information documenting a patient's health care services is considered the "patient health record." It includes all clinical or office records, all care, tests, and procedures done in health care or home care settings, as well as patient evaluations, and any participation in research or clinical databases. It's important that all medical records are organized and can be accessed by physicians, nurses, and other health care workers. A complete record gives a clear picture of a patient's medical condition as well as saves time and money by preventing duplication of laboratory tests and other procedures. It also allows medical billing workers to send appropriate bills to the patient or request reimbursement from insurance companies.

Great efforts have been made to organize and streamline the methods used by hospitals, clinics, and physicians' offices to gather and store patient records. At the center of this system are health information management specialists, who are key to the day-to-day operations of medical records departments.

At the start of every workday, health information management (HIM) specialists receive a request list from different physicians or departments of, say, a hospital or clinic. This list names every patient who will be seen that day—whether for an examination or follow-up, or perhaps for a blood test or x-ray. Other physicians may submit a list of patients needed for charting purposes or further research. Using this list, HIM specialists "pull" or electronically retrieve patients' records and deliver them to the appropriate physician or department.

Throughout the day, the medical records department will receive additional patient information from various sources, including off-site laboratories, hospitals, and physician's offices. This information could contain test results, physician consults, or a variety of other medical information. HIM specialists are responsible for coding any new diagnoses and incorporating new information into the patient's existing medical records.

As recently as 10 years ago, most medical records were in paper form, and a great deal of time was spent filing these papers into a patient's medical chart. Unfortunately medical records were sometimes misfiled due to human error. Today, most hospitals and clinics, and the majority of physician's offices, keep their medical records in an electronic format. Not only do electronic medical records reduce the chance for human error, they make it easier to quickly enter and obtain information. HIM specialists often attend training sessions to keep abreast of any new computer software applications or techniques to manage electronic medical records.

Some technicians are specially trained to work with medical coding. *Medical coders,* also known as *coding specialists,* transform medical diagnoses and procedures into a universally accepted set of numeral codes known as ICD-9-CM, which helps providers and insurance companies in their diagnosis and treatment of a disease, reimbursement, and surveillance of potential disease outbreaks. (The United States is scheduled to transition to a new coding system called ICD-10-CM on October 1, 2013.) This coded information is used by insurance companies or programs such as Medicare in the processing of claims.

Other technicians are specially trained to keep track of patients as they manage their illnesses. *Cancer registrars,* also known as *tumor registrars,* are needed to track information regarding patients and their fight against cancer. This information is used by researchers, health care professionals, and public policymakers to identify cancer groups, track treatment success, create cancer education programs, and support funding for additional treatment centers. Cancer registrars begin their work by creating a case file for every newly diagnosed patient in their assigned workplace, usually a hospital or cancer clinic. Information compiled includes the diagnosis of a cancerous or benign tumor, pathology reports, and medical reports. This first step will determine the patient's eligibility in the cancer registry. Next, cancer registrars abstract the case, or summarize the patient's medical records into standard coding used by the medical and research community. Specific coding is assigned to different data such as the patient's demographic, the type of cancer and its location, the stage of disease, and prescribed treatment details. Cancer registrars need to locate information and results from different locations, as patients are often sent to various physicians, clinics, and hospitals for various tests and procedures. Cancer registrars also conduct a yearly follow-up with each case, detailing any hospital admissions or changes in treatment as well as surveys from all attending physicians. Also important is the written follow-up with patients on how they have fared in the past year. All registry data is submitted to state cancer registries to identify high-risk groups, implement screening procedures, and give an estimated prognosis for many types of cancer.

Other HIM specialists work as *medical transcriptionists*. This is the process of taking handwritten notes or recorded evaluations and transforming them into an electronic format. Some hospitals and health care settings often outsource this duty, while others may keep it in-house. Transcription could mean simply keyboarding the physicians' notes, or finding and including the appropriate diagnosis or procedural code.

Health information administrators supervise health information management workers. They develop and implement policies that assure the appropriate storage and dissemination of health information.

Health information management specialists have other duties, including speaking with physicians or representatives from insurance companies, creating monthly work schedules, and ordering office supplies.

Full-time health information management specialists work about 40 hours a week, with opportunity for overtime. Those employed at hospitals or other health care facilities that offer round-the-clock care will have shift work.

HIM specialists work indoors in comfortable offices with cutting-edge computer technology. There may be separate areas for specific tasks such as file retrieval, transcription, coding, or quality review. Much of the work is detail oriented and done using a computer.

While they work in health care, HIM specialists (except cancer registrars) do not have any patient contact. However, they do interact with people from many different professions in order to clarify diagnoses or to obtain additional data.

REQUIREMENTS

HIGH SCHOOL

In high school, take courses in anatomy and physiology, biology, chemistry, mathematics (especially algebra), health, and computer science to prepare for the field.

POSTSECONDARY TRAINING

An associate's degree is typically required to enter the field, though some move into this field with work experience and on-the-job training. Health information administrators need at least a bachelor's degree.

The Commission on Accreditation for Health Informatics and Information Management Education accredits health information management programs. Visit its website, www.cahiim.org/accredpgms.asp, for a list of accredited programs. More than 200 programs are accredited by the Commission. Typical classes in a health information management program include Medical Terminology; Human Anatomy, Physiology, and Pathology; Health Data Management; Introduction to Pharmacology; Clinical Classification Systems; Clinical Data Analysis; Legal and Qualitative Aspects of Health Information; Principles of Health Information Management; Medical Reimbursement; Medical Transcription Practicum; Medical Coding Practicum; Medical Ethics; and Database Security and Management.

The American Health Information Management Association approves certificate programs in medical coding. Visit www.ahima.org/careers/college_search/search.aspx for a list of accredited programs. Sixty-nine percent of coders have some postsecondary training, according to a member survey from the AAPC; 18 percent have a bachelor's degree or higher.

CERTIFICATION AND LICENSING

Certification is offered by several professional associations, including the American Health Information Management Association, the AAPC, the Board of Medical Specialty Coding, the Association for Healthcare Documentation Integrity, the Professional Association of Healthcare Coding Specialists, the Practice Management Institute, the Institute of Certified Records Managers, and the National Cancer Registrars Association. Certification, while voluntary, is highly recommended. It is an excellent way to stand out from other job applicants and demonstrate your abilities to prospective employers.

OTHER REQUIREMENTS

Although the work is administrative in nature, HIM specialists must have a background in the health sciences, since accuracy and understanding of medical terminology are exceptionally important in these careers. They must translate physician notes, spot any inconsistencies, and avoid errors at all costs. Being detail oriented is a must for a career in health information management. Other important traits for HIM specialists include strong communication skills, the ability to work as a member of a team, and a willingness to continue to learn throughout one's career.

EXPLORING

There are many ways to learn more about a career as a health information management specialist. You can read books and journals (*Advance for Health Information Professionals,* www.advanceforhim.com) about the field, visit the websites of college health information management programs to learn about typical classes and possible career paths, and ask your teacher or school counselor to arrange an information interview with a HIM specialist. Professional associations can also provide information about the field. The American Health Information Management Association provides information on education and careers at its website, http://hicareers.com. You should also try to land a part-time job in a medical office. This will give you a chance to interact with HIM specialists and see if the career is a good fit for your abilities and interests.

EMPLOYERS

Approximately 277,700 medical records and health information technicians are employed in the United States. Nearly 40 percent are employed in hospitals. Other employers of HIM specialists include offices of physicians and other health care practitioners, outpatient clinics, surgical centers, nursing homes, managed-care facilities, home health agencies, pharmaceutical companies, long-term care facilities, state and federal government agencies that collect and disseminate health care information, and other health care facilities. Some HIM specialists are self-employed.

GETTING A JOB

Many health information management specialists obtain their first jobs as a result of contacts made through college internships, career fairs, or networking events. Others seek assistance in obtaining job leads from college career services offices, newspaper want ads, and employment websites. Additionally, professional associations, such as the American Health Information Management Association, the Association for Healthcare Documentation Integrity, the National Cancer Registrars Association, and the AAPC, provide job listings at their websites. See For More Information for contact information. *Advance for Health Information Professionals* also offers job listings for HIM specialists at its website, http://health-care-jobs.advanceweb.com. Medical transcriptionists can access job listings at MTJOBS (www.mtjobs.com). Those interested in positions with the federal government should visit the U.S. Office of Personnel Management's website, www.usajobs.opm.gov.

ADVANCEMENT

Health information management specialists advance by receiving pay raises and by earning bachelor's or master's degrees, which qualifies them to become health information managers. Those who obtain specialty certifications can become specialists such as medical transcriptionists.

EARNINGS

Median annual salaries for HIM specialists were $31,290 in 2009, according to the U.S. Department of Labor (USDL). Salaries ranged from less than $20,850 to $51,510 or more. The USDL reports the following mean annual earnings for HIM specialists by employer: federal executive branch, $45,120; general medical and surgical hospitals, $35,870; nursing care facilities, $33,100; outpatient care centers, $30,650; and offices of physicians, $28,460.

Medical transcriptionists earned salaries that ranged from less than $22,430 to $45,700 or more in 2009, according to the USDL. Those employed in general medical and surgical hospitals earned mean annual salaries of $34,480.

Employers offer a variety of benefits, including the following: medical, dental, and life insurance; paid holidays, vacations, and sick and personal days; 401(k) plans; profit-sharing plans; retirement and pension plans; and educational-assistance programs. Self-employed and part-time workers must provide their own benefits. Approximately 14 percent of HIM specialists are self-employed.

Health Care Career Resources on the Web

✔ *Career Guide to Industries: Healthcare* (www.bls.gov/oco/cg/cgs035.htm)

✔ Careers in Aging: Consider the Possibilities (www.careersinaging.com)

✔ DiscoverNursing.com (www.discovernursing.com)

✔ ExploreHealthCareers.org (http://explorehealthcareers.org)

✔ Health Professions (www.ama-assn.org/ama/pub/category/14598.html)

✔ HRSA Health Professions (http://bhpr.hrsa.gov)

EMPLOYMENT OUTLOOK

Employment for health information management specialists is expected to grow much faster than average for all careers through 2018, according to the U.S. Department of Labor (USDL). More opportunities are becoming available because of the increasing number of medical tests, procedures, and treatments that are being conducted and the federally mandated transition of paper medical records to electronic format. HIM specialists with a good knowledge of computer software and other technology will have the best job prospects.

Employment for medical transcriptionists is expected to grow about as fast as the average for all occupations through 2018. The USDL reports that "growing numbers of medical transcriptionists will be needed to amend patients' records, edit documents from speech recognition systems, and identify discrepancies in medical reports."

FOR MORE INFORMATION

For information on certification, contact the following organizations

AAPC
2480 South 3850 West, Suite B
Salt Lake City, UT 84120-7208
800-626-2633
info@aapc.com
www.aapc.com

ARMA International
11880 College Boulevard, Suite 450
Overland Park, KS 66210-1322
800-422-2762
www.arma.org

Association for Healthcare Documentation Integrity
4230 Kiernan Avenue, Suite 130
Modesto, CA 95356-9322
800-982-2182
ahdi@ahdionline.org
www.ahdionline.org

Practice Management Institute
9501 Console Drive, Suite 100
San Antonio, TX 78229-2033
800-259-5562
info@pmimd.com
www.pmimd.com

Professional Association of Healthcare Coding Specialists
218 East Bearss Avenue, #354
Tampa, FL 33613-1625

888-708-4707
info@pahcs.org
www.pahcs.org

For information on careers in health information management and accredited programs, contact
American Health Information Management Association
233 North Michigan Avenue,
21st Floor
Chicago, IL 60601-5809
312-233-1100
info@ahima.org
www.ahima.org

For a list of schools offering accredited programs, contact
Commission on Accreditation for Health Informatics and Information Management Education
233 North Michigan Avenue,
21st Floor
Chicago, IL 60601-5800
www.cahiim.org

To learn more about a career as a cancer registrar, contact
National Cancer Registrars Association
1340 Braddock Place, Suite 203
Alexandria, VA 22314-1651
703-299-6640
info@ncra-usa.org
www.ncra-usa.org

Interview: Claire Dixon-Lee

Claire Dixon-Lee, Ph.D., RHIA, CPH, FAHIMA is the executive director of the Commission on Accreditation for Health Informatics and Information Management Education (CAHIIM). She discussed the field of health information management with the editors of *Hot Health Care Careers*.

Q. **What is one thing that young people may not know about a career in health information management?**

A. The electronic health record and the impact of virtual health information transfer has opened many doors for health information professionals, from highly skilled technical jobs (associate-degree level) to foundational knowledge (baccalaureate level) and expanded leadership opportunities such as chief health information officer (graduate levels); the types of jobs and supporting industries (vendors, pharmaceuticals, public health, insurance companies, government, etc.) are many. Depending on what skill sets and interests each student brings to this field, the study of health information management (HIM) is the start of a career with endless opportunities.

Q.   What traits do quality HIM educational programs share? What should students look for when trying to choose a program?

A.   Students should look for CAHIIM-accredited programs or programs officially in CAHIIM Candidacy status, indicating that the institution and program is in the process of seeking CAHIIM accreditation. Students should look for institutions that are regionally or nationally accredited and participate in Title IV government student aid programs.

Programs are now emerging with a stronger focus in computer technology education; many are beginning to offer optional certificate tracks for specialized areas of study. Students should plan to seek the American Health Information Management Association professional entry-level certifications of registered health information technician (associate-degree level) and registered health information administrator (baccalaureate degree level), as well as post-baccalaureate options.

Q.   What are the most important personal and professional qualities for HIM professionals?

A.   HIM demonstrates a professional code of ethics—to protect the confidentiality and privacy of every patient's health information—thus practicing with integrity and dedication to improving health care through maintaining accurate and high-quality health information wherever it resides. At various levels, attention to detail, computer proficiency, strong biomedical studies (anatomy, physiology, and pathophysiology), understanding clinical work flows, the health care regulatory environment, legal issues, reimbursement rules, and supervisory/managerial abilities are highly important. Soft skills such as interpersonal communication ability, good written and oral communication skills, and desire for continuous learning and professionalism at every level are successful traits.

Q.   What is the employment outlook for HIM professionals? How is the field changing, and what should students do now to prepare for a successful career in the field?

A.   As mentioned earlier, greater technology advancements continue to evolve the profession, with traditional jobs changing and new jobs emerging in electronic health record implementation, training, and management; health information exchanges; physician group practices; long-term care and other non-acute care organizations; vendors; pharmaceutical firms; public health agencies; and within information technology departments in acute care, integrated delivery systems, and corporations.

To prepare for this career, in high school take courses in science, algebra, and computers; previous college or career change will require the biomedical sciences, computer literacy, and college math. Many options are available, including campus-based and online program offerings through various accredited colleges and universities. Recent government funding under the American Recovery and Reinvestment Act will make available short-term certificate programs. Many of these programs are found in conjunction with CAHIIM-accredited HIT and HIM programs around the country.

Visit www.hicareeers.com and www.cahiim.org for specific information on health information careers and CAHIIM accreditation.

Interview: Bryon Pickard

Bryon Pickard, MBA, RHIA is the director of operations for the Vanderbilt Medical Group Business Office in Nashville, Tennessee. He is also the past president of the American Health Information Management Association. Bryon discussed the field with the editors of *Hot Health Care Careers*.

Q. **What is one thing that young people may not know about a career in health information management?**

A. Ask this question a few years back, and you might hear a response that health information management is a well-kept secret. Believe me when I say this is definitely no longer the case.

Individuals need only look at the billions of dollars the federal government is pumping into meaningful use of EHR technology solutions over the next several years to realize that HIM is a vibrant and emerging career field. Trained professionals are needed not only to implement new systems, but to deal with the numerous activities and intricacies associated with managing and exchanging health information in a secure manner among providers, consumers, and the many other users of health information. The new American Recovery and Reinvestment Act and the Health Information Technology for Economic and Clinical Health Act "meaningful use" legislation guarantees investment toward expansion of this career field.

On the topic of legislation, the new Improper Payments Elimination and Recovery Act, which was signed into law recently, targets upwards of $110 billion in potential waste, fraud, and abuse. This directly impacts HIM professionals who bring to the table an understanding of clinical documentation requirements and implications necessary to ensure coding and billing integrity. Even more opportunities are on the horizon with upcoming transitions to new ANSI 5010 X12 standards and ICD-10-CM.

Q. **What are the most important personal and professional qualities for HIM professionals?**

A. Often the single most influential factor for a hiring decision or promotion is not just qualifications or experience, but rather behavioral characteristics and how much enthusiasm you generate. A couple more attributes to consider:

Plan Ahead: Be sure to write down where you want to be in five and 10 years, and then make it happen. Being able to visualize your future, and then documenting steps to get there, greatly increases the likelihood of succeeding.

Lifelong Learning: Successful HIM professionals are able to prove their worth every day and invest time to keep their skills fresh. Health care is going through dramatic change, and so are the skills needed to excel in HIM.

Commitment to You: Going the extra mile to do more than expected, along with enthusiasm and positive thinking, will yield career rewards. Also, take time to invest in yourself, gain the advice of a trusted mentor, and follow your instincts.

Q.   What is the employment outlook for HIM professionals? How is the field changing, and what should students do now to prepare for a successful career in the field?

A.   The sky is the limit for careers in health information management.

An already diverse collection of job titles and work settings is clearly escalating, particularly with the heightened pace of technology improvements. Let me be clear, though, it's not just the technology side of health information management, but rather the broader contributions of improving health and health care.

One of the biggest changes I foresee in the HIM field relates directly to the empowerment of consumers. As technical standards and information systems continue to evolve and become more uniform and user friendly, we can expect to see consumers increasingly utilize and interact with their own health information. This creates a whole new array of practice opportunities and job roles for health information management professionals.

To obtain a student perspective, I also asked Chartisha Maryland, HIM senior from Tennessee State University completing her professional practice here at Vanderbilt, how she is preparing for the future. Her response is right on target: "Be passionate about HIM, and grow your career by taking advantage of available HIM resources, attend professional conferences, volunteer, and network."

Sounds like very good advice to me!

LICENSED PRACTICAL NURSES

OVERVIEW

Licensed practical nurses (LPNs), also known as *licensed vocational nurses* in Texas and California, provide general health care to patients under the supervision of registered nurses and physicians. Their job duties depend largely on their work setting. To prepare for the field, LPNs must complete at least one year of postsecondary nursing training at a vocational or technical school or a community or junior college. Approximately 753,600 LPNs are employed in the United States. Employment opportunities are expected to be very good through 2018.

THE JOB

LPNs care for sick, injured, and disabled people. They handle a large share of the direct patient care in health care facilities today. They observe, record, and report changes in patients' conditions by taking patients' vital signs (blood pressure, pulse, respiration, temperature, height, and weight); administer medications and therapeutic treatments; and assist patients with bathing, dressing, and general personal hygiene. They help patients in and out of bed, dress wounds, and administer medication, taking careful note of the amount of the medication and the time it was administered and entering this information on patients' medical charts. They also note the patient's fluid intake and output. More and more today, these charts are now in electronic format.

LPNs must be comfortable using medical equipment such as IV lines, catheters, tracheotomy tubes, and respirators. For patients who need physical assistance, LPNs may help in getting them dressed and move about, or LPNs may assist them during mealtimes.

Most LPNs are generalists and are trained to work in any medical office setting, treating patients of all ages. Some specialize in a certain population, such as caring for the elderly in a nursing home or treating babies and young

FAST FACTS

High School Subjects
Biology
Chemistry

Personal Skills
Active listening
Communication
Critical thinking
Judgment and decision making

Minimum Education Level
Some postsecondary training

Salary Range
$28,000 to $39,000 to $55,000+

Employment Outlook
Much faster than the average

O*NET-SOC
29-2061.00

GOE
14.07.01

DOT
075

NOC
3233

children in a pediatric ward in a hospital. Experienced LPNs supervise nursing assistants and aides.

Regardless of where they work, LPNs play a critical role in gathering information about the patient and communicating it to other members of the patient's health care team. They ask the patient about his or her medical history, current symptoms, and any medications he or she might be taking. They monitor the patient for adverse reactions to newly prescribed medications or treatments and note changes in vital signs that may signal a problem. All this information is vital to help assist physicians and other specialists make diagnoses and prescribe treatments.

In addition to communicating with the patient's doctors and nurses, LPNs also spend time talking to the patient and his or her family about healthy living suggestions or how to care for a healing injury or newly diagnosed illness. They help make everyone more comfortable during a possibly scary time and try to answer any questions patients or family members may have.

Licensed practical nurses work in medical offices, hospitals, nursing homes, medical clinics, schools, and community health centers. Those who work in 24-hour settings such as hospitals may work evening or overnight shifts, and some LPNs work weekends or holidays. Since much of their work is physically demanding, LPNs must be in good shape. They help patients in and out of bed or move them to gurneys. They often bend, stoop, reach, and otherwise physically exert themselves during their shifts.

Like all health care workers, LPNs must follow standard procedures when caring for sick patients, such as wearing latex gloves or a mask and frequently washing their hands. While this career can be stressful and physically demanding at times, most LPNs view their careers as very rewarding.

REQUIREMENTS

HIGH SCHOOL

Take health, mathematics, biology, chemistry, physics, English, and speech in high school to prepare for a career in nursing.

POSTSECONDARY TRAINING

To become a LPN, you should attend a practical nurse training program at a technical or vocational school or a community college. Training lasts for approximately one year. Typical course work includes basic nursing concepts, anatomy, physiology, nutrition, first aid, nursing specialties (such as pediatric, obstetric, or gerontological nursing), and hands-on clinical experience. Visit Discover Nursing (www.discovernursing.com) for a database of nursing programs.

CERTIFICATION AND LICENSING

Certification, while not required, is an excellent way to demonstrate your nursing skills and expertise to potential employers. The National Association for Practical Nurse Education and Service offers specialty certification in pharmacology and long-term care. The National Federation of

Licensed Practical Nurses Education Foundation offers certification in IV therapy and gerontology. Contact these organizations for more information.

Nursing students need to pass the National Council Licensure Examination, or NCLEX-PN, in order to obtain licensure. The examination is administered by the National Council of State Boards of Nursing.

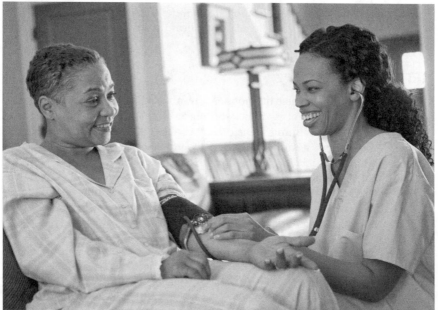

A licensed practical nurse takes a patient's blood pressure. (Jupiterimages/Thinkstock)

OTHER REQUIREMENTS

To be a successful LPN, you should have empathy for others, be decisive, enjoy working as a member of a team, be able to follow instructions (but also work independently, when necessary), have strong communication skills, and be willing to continue to learn throughout your career to keep your skills up to date.

EXPLORING

Read books and visit websites about nursing, talk with your counselor or teacher about setting up a presentation by a nurse, take a tour of a hospital or other health care setting, or volunteer at one of these facilities. Nursing websites, including those of professional associations, can also be a good source of information. Here are a few suggestions: Cybernurse.com (www.cybernurse.com), Discover Nursing (www.discovernursing.com), Nurse.com (www.nurse.com), and Futures in Nursing (http://futuresinnursing.org). You should also join Future Nurses organizations or student health clubs at your school.

EMPLOYERS

Approximately 753,600 LPNs are employed in the United States. Twenty-five percent work at hospitals, 28 percent in nursing care facilities, and 12 percent in offices of physicians. Others are employed by rehabilitation centers, home health care services, employment services, residential care facilities, nursing homes, and other health care facilities. Federal, state, and local government agencies employ licensed practical nurses. Opportunities can also be found in the U.S. military.

GETTING A JOB

Many LPNs obtain their first jobs as a result of contacts made through college clinical experiences or networking events. Others seek assistance in obtaining job leads from college career services offices, newspaper want ads, and employment websites. Additionally, professional associations, such as the National Association for Practical Nurse Education and Service and the National Federation of Licensed Practical Nurses, provide job listings at their websites. See For More Information for a list of organizations. Those interested in positions with the federal government should visit the U.S. Office of Personnel Management's website, www.usajobs.opm.gov.

ADVANCEMENT

Licensed practical nurses advance by receiving pay raises and becoming *charge nurses,* who supervise the work of other LPNs. Others become registered nurses by attending LPN-to-RN training programs. Some become nurse educators.

EARNINGS

Salaries for licensed practical nurses vary by type of employer, geographic region, and the worker's experience level and skills. Median annual salaries for LPNs were $39,820 in 2009, according to the U.S. Department of Labor (USDL). Salaries ranged from less than $28,890 to $55,090 or more. The USDL reports the following mean annual earnings for LPNs by employer: employment services, $46,190; nursing care facilities, $42,320; home health care services, $42,300; community care facilities for the elderly, $41,950; general medical and surgical hospitals, $39,980; and offices of physicians, $36,770.

Employers offer a variety of benefits, including the following: medical, dental, and life insurance; paid holidays, vacations, and sick days; personal days; 401(k) plans; profit-sharing plans; retirement and pension plans; and educational assistance programs. Self-employed workers must provide their own benefits.

EMPLOYMENT OUTLOOK

Employment for licensed practical nurses is expected to grow much faster than the average for all careers through 2018, according to the U.S. Department of

Labor. The growing population of people age 65 and over and increasing demand for health care services is creating excellent demand for licensed practical nurses. Employment opportunities will be strongest in nursing care facilities and home health care services. There is a shortage of nursing professionals in rural areas, which will create strong opportunities for those who are interested in working in and/or relocating to these and other underserved areas (such as inner cities).

Interview: David Schaefer

David Schaefer is a licensed practical nurse at Sharkey Issaquena Community Hospital in Rolling Fork, Mississippi. He discussed his career with the editors of *Hot Health Care Careers*.

FOR MORE INFORMATION

For information on certification and state boards of nursing, contact
National Association for Practical Nurse Education and Service
1940 Duke Street, Suite 200
Alexandria, VA 22314-3452
703-933-1003
www.napnes.org

For information on licensing, contact
National Council of State Boards of Nursing
111 East Wacker Drive, Suite 2900
Chicago, IL 60601-4277
312-525-3600
info@ncsbn.org
www.ncsbn.org

For information about certification, contact
National Federation of Licensed Practical Nurses
605 Poole Drive
Garner, NC 27529-5203
919-779-0046
www.nflpn.org

Q.   What made you want to enter this career?

A.   I always knew I wanted to be a nurse. I loved helping people, and what better way to do that than being a nurse?

Q.   Can you tell us about your workplace?

A.   Sharkey Issaquena Community Hospital operates 20 acute, observation, swingbed, and long-term care beds and also has a 10-bed geriatric psychiatric unit. LPNs have to be EMT-Basic certified at this facility; we are the primary ambulance riders.

Q.   Can you please briefly describe a day in your life on the job?

A.   In the hospital setting, LPNs have a lot of direct patient care. A normal work day for me goes something like this: my day starts around 6:30 P.M. Usually report is over shortly after 7 P.M., depending on the patient load. At that time we observe the patients and collect our data for our opening notes. We check the carts for changes in the plan of care along with possible medicine changes, lab work and/or results, or diet changes. It's around 8 P.M. at this time, and medicines are due. Throughout the night patients are observed and monitored every two hours. It's finally 6 A.M. and we start gathering data for our closing notes, such as daily weights, fasting blood glucose levels, tallying output/intake for the total shift. Also at this time, any morning medications that have to be given before breakfast are given. It's 7 A.M., and it's time to report off to the oncoming shift.

Q.   What are the most important personal and professional qualities for licensed practical nurses?

A.   The most personal quality is having respect for all patients and their families. One must put himself or herself in the shoes of the patient or their families to correctly care for the patient. Being committed to your job as a nurse is a major professional quality. No patient ever wants a nurse who is only halfway doing his or her job.

Q.   What are some of the pros and cons of your job?

A.   Some pros of my job include helping to restore the health of the patient, giving hope in a hopeless situation, and also the week I have off. Cons of the job include long work hours and the death of patients, just to include a few.

Q.   What advice would you give to young people who are interested in the field? What are the best ways to find a job?

A.   I tell people who are considering becoming a nurse that you have to have compassion and empathy, and you have to be willing to care for your patients and sometimes their families. Nurses can't work for just the salary alone, they have to enjoy their jobs because if not, the quality of care given is terrible.

Some of the best ways to find a job are to market oneself and always be willing to help out. Instead of creating a problem, create a solution.

Q.   What is the employment outlook for LPNs?

A.   For years now, the rumor has been that LPNs are going to all be replaced by RNs. My reply to that is that the nursing industry cannot survive without the help of LPNs. Why on earth would you hire an all-RN staff when you could hire several LPNs and hire more people? LPNs are here to stay. LPNs are real NURSES, and we give awesome care to our patients.

MEDICAL ASSISTANTS

OVERVIEW

Medical assistants perform administrative and clinical duties at medical offices, hospitals, inpatient/outpatient clinics, nursing homes, and long-term care facilities, and in other health care settings. Their duties include taking patients' medical histories, assisting physicians during procedures, conducting simple tests, updating patients' files in electronic databases, and completing paperwork. Some medical assistants have specialized duties based on the size or type of practice. There are no formal education requirements for medical assistants. Some learn their skills via on-the-job training; many train for the field by completing postsecondary programs that last one or two years. Approximately 483,600 medical assistants are employed in the United States. Opportunities for medical assistants are expected to be excellent through 2018.

FAST FACTS

High School Subjects
Biology
Mathematics

Personal Skills
Following instructions
Helping
Technical

Minimum Education Level
High school diploma

Salary Range
$20,000 to $28,000 to $46,000+

Employment Outlook
Much faster than the average

O*NET-SOC
31-9092.00

GOE
14.02.01

DOT
079

NOC
6631

THE JOB

Medical assistants work under the supervision of physicians, nurses, and managers. Many of their duties are administrative in nature. These include checking in patients, answering the phone, sorting mail, and scheduling appointments. *Administrative medical assistants* also maintain medical records, file patient records, and complete requests for insurance reimbursement. Some are trained to perform monthly insurance electronic billing for services rendered as well as to send out monthly statements and record payments that are received. Others are specially trained to perform medical transcription (the written or typed transcription of a doctor's recorded notes).

Clinical medical assistants have some administrative duties but largely focus on helping the doctor before, during, and after patient examinations and procedures. Before bringing a patient to the examination room, clinical medical assistants prepare the room, making sure the examination table is clean and supplies and instruments are ready for use. They then take the patient's pulse, blood pressure, and temperature; measure his or her weight; and talk with the patient regarding the nature of his or her visit and any complaints about health or symptoms, writing this information down for review by the physician. They assist the physician during examinations and certain procedures by handing instruments to the physician or readying medications or supplies for use. After each procedure, clinical medical assistants dispose of contaminated supplies and sterilize equipment and instruments. Some clinical medical assistants are trained to remove sutures, change dressings and bandages, collect specimens, or administer injections. They also operate diagnostic equipment such as electrocardiogram or x-ray machines. As directed by a physician, clinical medical assistants also help patients arrange for hospital admission, give needed orders for laboratory work, pass along physician referrals, and give instruction to patients regarding new prescriptions, special diets, or additional treatments.

Some medical assistants have specialized duties specific to their workplace. For example, *podiatric medical assistants* are trained to make castings of feet, take x-rays of the feet or ankle, and assist the podiatrist during surgeries.

Optometric medical assistants and *ophthalmic medical assistants* have special duties related to care and health of the eyes. They conduct tests such as a lensometry (which measures for proper lens prescription) or tonometry (which determines fluid pressure, a sign of glaucoma). They also conduct other tests to measure visual acuity or eye muscle function. Some administer drops to dilate the eye in preparation for an exam or administer other medicinal drops. Ophthalmic medical assistants also educate patients about the proper care and insertion of contact lenses.

Medical assistants work in well-lit, clean offices. Full-time medical assistants work 40 hours a week, with some evening or weekend hours required. There is no official uniform, but most medical assistants choose to wear medical scrubs or smocks with pants. Comfortable shoes are a must, since medical assistants are on their feet for a good part of the day. Medical assistants often use gloves, masks, or other protective gear, especially when assisting physicians with procedures or handling spent syringes or needles.

REQUIREMENTS

HIGH SCHOOL

Take health and science classes in high school—especially anatomy, physiology, biology, and chemistry. English and speech classes will help you develop your writing skills, which you will use frequently during your workday. Since medical professionals are increasingly using computers to record and store data about patients, computer science classes (especially those involving database management) will be useful. If you attend a vocational high school, you might be able to take medical-assisting classes or even participate in a formal training program to prepare for the field.

POSTSECONDARY TRAINING

There are no formal education requirements for medical assistants. Some learn their skills via on-the-job training; many train for the field by completing postsecondary programs that last one or two years. Some of the topics covered in medical-assisting classes include anatomy, physiology, medical terminology, clinical and diagnostic procedures, pharmaceutical principles, laboratory techniques, first aid, medical ethics, and office skills (such as keyboarding, recordkeeping, transcription, accounting, and insurance processing). Students also complete an internship at a medical office as part of their studies.

The Accrediting Bureau of Health Education Schools and the Commission on Accreditation of Allied Health Education Programs accredit medical-assisting programs. The Commission on Accreditation of Ophthalmic Medical Programs accredits ophthalmic medical-assisting programs. See the For More Information section for contact information for these organizations.

CERTIFICATION AND LICENSING

Certification is offered by several associations, including the American Association of Medical Assistants, the Association of Medical Technologists, and the National Healthcareer Association. Specialty certification is available from the American Society of Podiatric Medical Assistants and the Joint Commission on Allied Health Personnel in Ophthalmology. Certification, while voluntary, is highly recommended. It is an excellent way to stand out from other job applicants and demonstrate your abilities to prospective employers.

OTHER REQUIREMENTS

Medical assistants interact with patients, physicians, nurses, and other health care professionals throughout the day, so it's important that you be able to get along with many different types of personalities and work as a member of a team. You should also be organized and work well under pressure, especially when work is busy and you are asked to perform multiple tasks or handle multiple assistants. Other important traits include the ability to follow instructions, compassion, and manual dexterity and good vision.

EXPLORING

There are many ways to learn more about a career as a medical assistant. You can read books and magazines (such as *CMA Today*, www.aama-ntl.org/CMAToday) about the field, visit the websites of college medical assisting programs to learn about typical classes and possible career paths, and ask your teacher or school counselor to arrange an information interview with a medical assistant. Professional associations can also provide information about the field. The American Association of Medical Assistants provides a wealth of information on medical assistants and careers at its website, www.aama-ntl.org. Try to land a part-time job in a medical office. This will give you a chance to interact with medical assistants and see if the career is a good fit for your interests and abilities.

EMPLOYERS

Approximately 483,600 medical assistants are employed in the United States. About 62 percent work in offices of physicians. Thirteen percent work at public and private hospitals, and 11 percent work in offices of other health practitioners, such as optometrists, podiatrists, and chiropractors. Others are employed at outpatient care centers and residential care facilities.

GETTING A JOB

Many medical assistants obtain their first jobs as a result of contacts made through college internships, career fairs, or networking events. Others seek assistance in obtaining job leads from college career services offices, newspaper want ads, and employment websites. Additionally, professional associations, such as the Association of Technical Personnel in Ophthalmology, provide job listings at their websites. See For More Information for a list of organizations. Those interested in positions with the federal government should visit the U.S. Office of Personnel Management's website, www.usajobs.opm.gov.

ADVANCEMENT

With further education, medical assistants can become nurses, physician assistants, physicians, or health sciences professors. Administrative medical assistants can become office managers or work in other managerial positions.

EARNINGS

Salaries for medical assistants vary by type of employer, geographic region, and the worker's experience, education, and skill level. Median annual salaries for medical assistants were $28,650 in 2009, according to the U.S. Department of Labor (USDL). Salaries ranged from less than $20,750 to $39,970 or more. The USDL reports the following mean annual earnings for medical assistants by employer: psychiatric and substance abuse hospitals, $46,430; offices of dentists, $35,920; scientific research and development services, $33,810; local government, $31,900; colleges, universities, and professional schools, $30,850; general medical and surgical hospitals, $30,830; outpatient care centers, $29,830; offices of physicians, $29,810; offices of other health practitioners, $26,490.

The American Association of Medical Assistants reports that certified medical assistants earned average annual salaries of $31,361 in 2010. Medical assistants with 0-2 years of experience earned average salaries of $25,034. Those with 16 or more years of experience earned $35,862.

Medical assistants usually receive benefits such as health and life insurance, vacation days, sick leave, and a savings and pension plan. Part-time workers must provide their own benefits.

EMPLOYMENT OUTLOOK

Employment for medical assistants is expected to grow by 34 percent from 2008 to 2018, according to the U.S. Department of Labor—making it one of the fastest-growing occupations in the nation. Factors that are fueling growth include the increasing U.S. population (especially the elderly, who typically need more medical care than other demographic groups), technological advances that are allowing people to live longer, the increasing number of medical facilities that need support staff such as medical assistants, and the increasing prevalence of certain diseases and conditions, such as diabetes and obesity, which will create demand for more support staff to help treat patients. Opportunities wil be best for those with formal training and certification.

FOR MORE INFORMATION

For information on accreditation, contact
Accrediting Bureau of Health Education Schools
7777 Leesburg Pike, Suite 314-North
Falls Church, VA 22043-2411
www.abhes.org

For information on careers, earnings, and certification, contact
American Association of Medical Assistants
20 North Wacker Drive, Suite 1575
Chicago, IL 60606-2963
www.aama-ntl.org

For certification information, contact
American Medical Technologists
10700 West Higgins Road
Park Ridge, IL 60018-3707
www.amt1.com

For information on career options for optometric medical assistants, contact
American Optometric Association
243 North Lindbergh Boulevard
Creve Coeur, MO 63141-7881
www.aoa.org

For information on careers in podiatric medical assisting, contact
American Society of Podiatric Medical Assistants
www.aspma.org

For information on careers in ophthalmic medical assisting, contact
Association of Technical Personnel in Ophthalmology
2025 Woodlane Drive
St. Paul, MN 55125-2998
www.atpo.org

For information on accredited programs, contact
Commission on Accreditation of Allied Health Education Programs
1361 Park Street
Clearwater, FL 33756-6039
www.caahep.org

For information on accredited programs, contact
Commission on Accreditation of Ophthalmic Medical Programs
2025 Woodlane Drive
St. Paul, MN 55125-2998
www.jcahpo.org/CoA-OMP/about

For information on certification, contact the following organizations
Joint Commission on Allied Health Personnel in Ophthalmology
2025 Woodlane Drive
St. Paul, MN 55125-2998
www.jcahpo.org

National Healthcareer Association
7500 West 160th Street
Stilwell, KS 66085-8100
www.nhanow.com

Interview: Lisa Lee

Lisa Lee is a medical assistant at Tanner Clinic in Layton, Utah. She is also a trustee of the American Association of Medical Assistants. Lisa discussed her career with the editors of *Hot Health Care Careers*.

Q. Can you tell us about the Tanner Clinic? How long have you worked in the field? What made you want to enter this career?

A. Tanner Clinic is a large multi-specialty clinic with 70+ physicians as well as in-house lab, magnetic resonance imaging, computed tomography, and radiology. We also have a couple of surgery suites where minor procedures are performed, and we do all our billing in-house as well. I have worked at Tanner Clinic for 17 years, all for the same orthopedic surgeon, and in addition to my regular job I'm the supervisor of the orthopedic department. Prior to coming to Tanner Clinic, I worked for a plastic surgeon in his private office for nine years, so I have worked in the field for 26 years.

I entered this field primarily because of the example of my mother. She is also a certified medical assistant and has worked in the field for more than 50 years, all of them at the same clinic. I watched her while I was growing up and saw firsthand the compassion she had for her patients and admired the service she provided for them. After I completed college with a bachelor's degree in sociology I discovered I wasn't going to enjoy working in that environment, so I thought more about my mom's example and decided to look into the medical field. I have been there ever since.

Q. What is one thing that young people may not know about a career as a medical assistant?

A. I think one of the main things that young people may not know is that medical assisting is hard work, physically as well as emotionally. At least in our clinic, the job goes way beyond greeting a patient at the reception desk or walking them back to an exam room. Sometimes we push their wheelchairs back to the exam rooms, and sometimes we have to assist these patients up on to the exam tables. We are in constant motion running specimens to the lab, walking patients to radiology, fitting braces and splints, etc. Emotionally we see patients at their best and their worst. When someone is in pain or confused, it is not uncommon for them to lash out at the first available person, which is often the medical assistant. We have to just know that it is not us they are yelling at. We have to make decisions constantly as to the priority of the things we are being asked to do, and those decisions do not always make all parties happy. All this aside, I will say that there is no greater profession, in my mind. All the hard work pays off with the satisfaction that I get out of seeing a patient's smile after helping them or from hearing even one patient say thank you. I love my job and would not want to trade professions.

Q. Can you please briefly describe a day in your life on the job?

A. No two days are alike, but typically I arrive before my doctor and make sure the computers are up and ready to go, and then I return any phone calls that have come in since the last time we were in the office. At our clinic we are hired to work for just one doctor and do everything that is required in his/her practice. We are not assigned to just one particular task such as phlebotomy or loading the patients into an exam room and taking their vitals and their histories.

A certified medical assistant is described as being highly trained and multi-skilled, and I use every one of those skills I was trained in almost every day. During the course of any given day I answer all incoming phone calls and am responsible for taking care of any actions derived from those calls. This includes calling in prescription refills and juggling the schedule sometimes and, of course, documenting all calls in the EMR (electronic medical record). I obtain prior authorizations from insurance companies for office procedures as well as for outside surgeries. I also schedule these surgeries at the appropriate facilities. I take care of the hospital billings as well. All of the above is what I do inbetween patients or while the doctor is with the patient. Additionally, I apply and remove all casts, change dressings, remove sutures, apply braces and splints, perform blood draws when directed, and administer all injections other than intra-articular injections. I load the exam rooms and take the histories and record the vitals of the patients. I schedule any radiology exams that the doctor orders and instruct the patients if there are any requirements for their exams. When my doctor gives an intra-articular injection or performs minor surgery in our clinic, I do the prep for the procedure as well.

Q. What are the most important personal and professional qualities for people in your career?

A. I think you need to honestly like people. It is important to be happy and to smile. Smiles are contagious and can make people feel at ease. If you are not a people person, medical assisting may not be the best career. I think most people are friendly, and I love interacting with our patients and really getting to know them. I try to learn little things about them or their families, and when they come in the next time and I remember those things, the patients really light up. Sometimes this small act makes their day, and I've made a friend for life. I also feel a medical assistant needs to have true compassion for and genuinely care for the patients he or she serves. This makes all the difference in the world for the experience those patients have with the doctor you work for. The medical assistant can make or break the relationship.

It is important to remember that in the medical field we deal with people from all walks of life. No one is offended by professionalism, but many are offended by the lack of it. As a medical assistant, you should remember that you represent the profession as a whole, and it is very important how you look to the public. Wild and crazy hair styles, excessive jewelry or nails, or some of the other fashion trends that are popular are out of place in the physician's office. This sometimes makes the patients feel uncomfortable, and if they are not comfortable they don't very often return. It is also important to make sure we wear uniforms that are clean and pressed. We don't want to look like we woke up and just threw something on. We need to look professional and act professional at all times, and this includes how we speak.

Foul language or slang has no place in a medical office, and even beyond that (which should be obvious), we need to make sure we speak using proper grammar. The public assumes we are professionals in all aspects of the word and that we are well educated, and it only takes one slip to change their perception of that.

Q. What are some of the pros and cons of your job?

A.   The pros of my job are easy. It is very rewarding to see someone come into the office in pain or scared and have them leave more comfortable and happy and know that I had a part in that outcome, especially when it comes to the kids. I love working with kids. There is nothing false about a child. You know when they are hurting and when they are better, and they always have a true desire to get better. Their smiles are the best. I also love the satisfaction of a job well done. I very much enjoy interacting with the patients and getting to know them. I have some very special friendships that have come about because of my job. I love the smiles, and the pats on the back, and the hugs, and the thank-yous. We have one patient who tells me every time she comes in that I'm a "special person" and she "loves" me, and those kinds of comments make my day even when it's been a bad day. I just love my job and, once again, the feeling of satisfaction I get from a job well done is indescribable.

The cons of my job are much harder to define because I don't know that I really think there are any, other than the occasional grumpy patient. About the only things I could come up with that would be considered cons are the wages and the work schedule I have. Taking into account the enormous amount of responsibility and sometimes the liability a medical assistant has, the wages we are paid are not very good, and I believe the pay must improve in order to attract more people to the profession. I think this is slowly beginning to change, as employers are seeing the value of hiring certified medical assistants and are recognizing the asset we are to the offices we work for, but we are not paid very well right now. The work schedule is not very flexible either. I am responsible to be at work when my doctor is at work, and this does not always fit in with the schedule my family may have, or my dentist, or anyone else I may need to schedule an appointment with. If I have sick kids or need a day off for some other reason, I can't just call in sick and figure I can catch up the next day. It is my responsibility to find my own coverage if I am unable to fill my shift. At Tanner Clinic we all help each other out and cover for one another if our doctor is out of the office and we need a day off, but finding coverage can be a problem at times. Another thing about the schedule is that I don't have a 9 to 5 job. I may get to work at 9:00, but I don't leave until the last patient has left and all the paperwork has been completed. This may be 5:00, but most of the time it is more like 7:00. For me, I don't mind the long days because the job is so rewarding and I have a very understanding family, but the schedule can be a con.

Q. What advice would you give to young people who are interested in the field?

A.   I would tell them that where they go to school is very important. They should research the schools they are interested in attending and make sure the school they select is accredited by CAAHEP (Committee on

Accreditation of Allied Health Education Programs) or ABHES (Accrediting Bureau of Health Education Schools). Young people (or older people, for that matter) should not look for the program they can complete the quickest, they should look for the program that will give them the best education and best prepare them to work with the public and the fast-paced nature of the medical-assisting profession. CAAHEP and ABHES programs provide this training. The programs are more intense and take longer to complete, but upon completion of the program and successfully taking the certification exam they will earn the certified medical assistant (CMA) credential, which is the gold standard of medical-assisting credentials. Some of the other schools will try to convince students the credential they offer is just as good as the CMA credential, but that is not correct. Some credentials are valid only in the states where they were earned, and some credentials are not even recognized by employers. The CMA credential is a national certification and is good in all states. So, my best advice would be that the education portion of the profession matters a great deal and potential students should make sure that if they are going to invest the time and the money they should get the best bang for their buck, which is the CMA credential.

Interview: Tina Del Buono

Tina Del Buono, PMAC, XT is a podiatric medical assistant and office manager at Santa Rosa Foot and Ankle Associates in Santa Rosa, California. She is also the director of intra-professional relations at the American Society of Podiatric Medical Assistants. She discussed her career and the field of medical assisting with the editors of *Hot Health Care Careers*.

Q. How long have you worked in the field? What made you want to enter this career?

A. I have worked here in the office for 14 years. I was a medical transcriptionist who was doing the transcription for this facility and found this specialty very interesting. They had a part-time opening, and I applied. I started as a back office assistant and then learned all aspects of the practice. I now am the office manager.

Q. What is one thing that young people may not know about a career as a podiatric medical assistant?

A. One of the great things about working in podiatry is that you can learn under your physician's guidance. You can study and take a national certification exam in either administrative assisting or clinical or both. Keeping people on their feet is very rewarding and a key to them staying healthy.

Q. Can you please briefly describe a day in your life on the job?

A. I am crossed trained, as a lot of podiatric medical assistants are. I work front and back office as needed. We start at 8 A.M. with patients. I will take patients to the treatment rooms and help them with their shoes and socks if needed. Taking the subjective part of the chart note is important for the physician, as he or she then can see what the patients' problems are or how they have been since their last appointment. Interacting with patients is one of the best parts of our job. Being able to listen to the problems they present with and getting the necessary information down for the doctor can be a challenge at times. Learning how to communicate with the patients to enhance the care that they will receive is very reward-ing. Making the visit run smoothly and efficiently is a big part of what we do, and that means understanding what my doctor may need and having it ready for him/her when he/she enters the room with the patient. After the patient leaves, it is our job to clean and prepare the room for the next patient. When helping in the front office we check in patients, collect their balance or copayment, and obtain any necessary paperwork that we may need. Again, communication skills are probably one of the most important skills we need in our job as a medical assistant. We may also post insurance payments, call insurance companies for our payments, and work collections and billing.

Q.   What are some of the pros and cons of your job?

A.   Pros: Helping people to feel better by knowing that I worked with the doc-tor to make that happen. Whether we are in the room with the patient or the one who makes sure they have the proper insurance benefits for the doctor to proceed with treatment, we are part of making their treatment happen. [I like] seeing patients who have bad wounds or broken bones get better and knowing that our interactions with them were caring and pro-fessional. There is nothing better than helping people to feel better.

Cons: In today's medical world we have a lot of issues with all the different insurance companies, and patients get frustrated and angry with us instead of with their insurance companies.

Q.   What advice would you give to young people who are interested in the field? What's the best way to land a job?

A.   First of all, whatever specialty you might be interested in make sure you investigate what part of the body it deals with, because in podiatry you need to like feet and have to be able to touch people's feet. Read as much as you can about the field, research it on the Internet. There is so much information about podiatry, and the more you know the better it will be when you apply for a podiatric assisting job. Call the podiatry offices in your area and see if you can shadow the assistants there for a few days so you can see what they do to better understand how podiatric medical offices function and what types of problems they deal with.

MEDICAL SCIENTISTS

OVERVIEW

Medical scientists work to enhance and prolong human life by conducting research on human diseases and conditions. Their research has resulted in advances in the diagnosis, treatment, and prevention of many diseases and conditions. Medical scientists need a Ph.D. in a biological science; some scientists also have medical degrees. Approximately 109,400 medical scientists work in the United States. Employment in the field is expected to be good through 2018.

THE JOB

The invention of the airplane has made even the remotest reaches of the world accessible. One can fly from the United States to Africa in the better part of a day. However, that new freedom comes with a price. Infectious diseases can also travel the globe via airplane, bringing illnesses such as malaria or yellow fever to populations that have not experienced these diseases in decades. Thankfully we have vaccines for many of these diseases, which has stopped their large-scale spread. We can thank medical scientists for these and other discoveries that help protect our health.

FAST FACTS
High School Subjects Biology Chemistry Mathematics
Personal Skills Communication Complex problem solving Critical thinking Scientific Technical
Minimum Education Level Doctorate degree (medical scientists, except epidemiologists) Master's degree (epidemiologists)
Salary Range $40,000 to $74,000 to $138,000+
Employment Outlook Much faster than the average (medical scientists, except epidemiologists) Faster than the average (epidemiologists)
O*NET-SOC 19-1041.00, 19-1042.00
GOE 02.03.01
DOT 041
NOC 2121, 3111

Most medical scientists specialize in a particular discipline. For example, *pharmacologists* study the effects of drugs on biological systems; *cytologic scientists* study cellular materials; *histologic scientists* study tissue structure; and *medical microbiologists* work to identify the microorganisms that cause disease or can be used to fight illness. *Epidemiologists* investigate the causes and spread of disease and try to prevent or control disease outbreaks. *Research epidemiologists* study diseases in the field and in medical laboratories to find ways to prevent future outbreaks. *Applied epidemiologists* respond to disease outbreaks. They find out what caused the outbreak and suggest ways to contain it. They typically work for state health agencies. *Infectious disease specialists* help physicians and public health workers identify diseases that are difficult to diagnose, are accompanied by a high fever, or do not respond to treatment.

Most medical scientists work in laboratories, preparing samples to study cell structure or studying bacteria or other organisms. They may examine tissues, cells, or microorganisms, often using an electron microscope. Some analyze changes in cells that signal health problems. Medical scientists must understand the behavior of a healthy cell to help diagnose a sick or dying cell. Similarly, they take note of the effects of certain treatments on cells to fine-tune drugs. Medical scientists also try to find ways to prevent health problems. For example, they may study the link between radiation from x-rays and cancer or between alcoholism and liver disease.

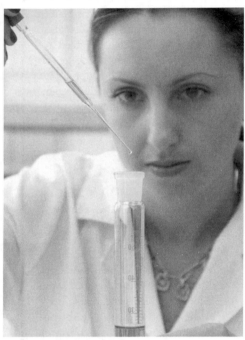

Once they finish collecting data, medical scientists use statistical modeling software and other computer-based technologies to analyze their findings. Then they write reports or articles about their findings. Depending on where they work, scientists

A medical scientist studies a sample in a laboratory. (Thinkstock)

may also make presentations on their research or write articles for publication in scientific journals.

In hospitals and medical offices, medical scientists conduct tests on blood and tissue samples to diagnosis illnesses. They send their results to *physicians,* who then decide on treatment options. Some medical scientists are also physicians. These individuals interact with patients directly. They administer new or experimental drug treatments to patients, closely monitoring their health during trials. They adjust dosage levels to minimize potential negative side effects or increase levels to maximize the medicine's effectiveness.

Some medical scientists work for pharmaceutical companies. They work to create new drugs or improve existing ones that are manufactured by their employer. The downside to working in business is these scientists are sometimes limited to the business goals of their company.

A field that has taken off in recent years is biomedical research. *Biomedical scientists* study genetics and DNA to pinpoint their relationship to well-being or illnesses. Biomedical breakthroughs have made it possible to manufacture human substances such as insulin that have improved the lives of millions diagnosed with diabetes. Biomedical scientists hope to apply this same approach to discover the genetic causes of cancers, Alzheimer's disease, and Parkinson's disease, among other diseases.

Medical scientists also do a lot of writing for their job, either mapping out their research approach before they begin their lab work or writing about their end results. They prepare their findings for publication or simply to share with their colleagues and other scientists. Many scientists depend on grant money to conduct their work, so much of their time is spent writing detailed proposals to continue or increase their funding sources. The National Institutes of Health administers many of these grants, and competition for funding is intense. The better that medical scientists can convey the goals of their proposed study, the better their chances of securing a grant.

Medical scientists also do a considerable amount of reading. In order to enhance their own work, they must understand the discoveries and failures that came before them. The field of medical science changes every day, so they must stay on top of the latest breakthroughs.

Most scientists work in laboratories, hunched over a microscope, research article, or computer. Eyestrain and physical stress involved in being stationary for many hours at a time is part of the job. The stereotype of a lone scientist in a dark and dingy lab is not usually accurate. Medical scientists often work with teams of scientists, research subjects, engineers, doctors, and other medical professionals in their work. Because their work can expose them to infectious diseases, medical scientists must follow strict guidelines in the handling of hazardous materials. They often wear a lab coat and may also wear goggles, gloves, and face masks or respirators depending on their work.

Since research funding is often obtained through the awarding of grant money, scientists face the stress of deadlines for applying or, once they receive a grant, reporting results to the grantor agency. Medical scientists typically work standard 9 to 5 hours, but weekend and evening hours may be required when working on certain experiments or projects. The U.S. Department of Labor reports that research and development professionals worked an average of 36.8 hours per week in 2008—approximately 3.2 hours more than workers in all private industries.

REQUIREMENTS

HIGH SCHOOL

In high school, take as many health, biology, anatomy and physiology, mathematics, biology, chemistry, physics, English, and speech classes in high school as possible.

POSTSECONDARY TRAINING

Medical scientists need a Ph.D. in a biological science; some scientists also have medical degrees. A growing number of new graduates also complete postdoctoral work in the laboratory of a senior researcher. Epidemiologists need at least a master's degree in public health, although some employers require a doctorate or a medical degree.

To prepare for graduate study, you should earn a bachelor's degree in a biological science. Biology-related degrees are offered by thousands of colleges and universities throughout the United States.

Once students have earned their bachelor's degrees, the U.S. Department of Labor reports that "there are two main paths for prospective medical scientists. They can enroll in a university Ph.D. program in the biological sciences; these programs typically take about six years of study, and students specialize in one particular field, such as genetics, pathology, or bioinformatics. They can also enroll in a joint M.D.-Ph.D. program at a medical college; these programs typically take seven to eight years of study, where students learn both the clinical skills needed to be a physician and the research skills needed to be a scientist." Visit www.aamc.org/students/considering/exploring_medical/research/mdphd to learn more about M.D.-Ph.D. dual degree training.

The American Society for Pharmacology and Experimental Therapeutics offers a list of graduate-level pharmacology training programs at its website, www.aspet.org/training_programs.

CERTIFICATION AND LICENSING

The American Board of Clinical Pharmacology (www.abcp.net) offers voluntary board certification to pharmaceutical scientists. The Certification Board of Infection Control and Epidemiology (www.cbic.org), a subgroup of the Association for Professionals in Infection Control and Epidemiology, offers voluntary certification to epidemiologists. Contact these organizations for more information.

The USDL reports that "medical scientists who administer drug or gene therapy to human patients, or who otherwise interact medically with patients—drawing blood, excising tissue, or performing other invasive procedures—must be licensed physicians." To become licensed, physicians must pass a licensing examination, graduate from an accredited medical school, and complete one to seven years of graduate medical education.

OTHER REQUIREMENTS

Medical scientists should have strong scientific and research skills. They must be extremely focused in order to conduct meticulous, time-consuming research that may or may not result in ground-breaking discoveries. Medical scientists need to be excellent communicators. They frequently convey their findings to colleagues, the press, and the general public in both oral and written format. They also need to have good writing skills in order to craft grant proposals that help them obtain funding for their research. Other important traits include strong organizational skills, the ability to work independently or as part of a team, and an interest in continuing to learn and stay abreast of industry developments throughout their careers.

EXPLORING

There are many ways to learn more about a career as a medical scientist. You can read books and journals about medical scientific research and visit the websites of college programs that offer degrees in pharmacology, genetics, biology, biotechnology, biomedical science, and related fields, and you can ask your teacher or school counselor to arrange an information interview with a medical scientist. Professional associations can also provide information about the field. For example, the American Association of Pharmaceutical Scientists offers videos and interviews with scientists at its website, www.aaps.org/features/10Questions. The American Society for Pharmacology and Experimental Therapeutics provide information on pharmacology and careers at its website, www.aspet.org. The Infectious Diseases Society of America offers *A World of Opportunities: Career Paths in Infectious Diseases and HIV Medicine* at its website, www.idsociety.org. The Association of American Medical Colleges provides information about a career in biomedical research at its website, www.aamc.org/students.

EMPLOYERS

Approximately 109,400 medical scientists are employed in the United States. Medical scientists work for universities, government agencies, medical offices, nonprofit research organizations, and hospitals, and in the private sector for pharmaceutical companies. The U.S. Department of Labor reports that "about 31 percent of medical scientists were employed in scientific research and development services firms; another 27 percent were employed in educational services; 13 percent were employed in pharmaceutical and medicine manufacturing; and 10 percent were employed in hospitals." Although opportunities are available throughout the United States, more than half of all research and development workers are employed in seven states: California, Illinois, Maryland, Massachusetts, New Jersey, New York, and Pennsylvania.

GETTING A JOB

Many medical scientists obtain their first jobs as a result of contacts made through postdoctoral positions. Others seek assistance in obtaining job leads from college career services offices, networking events, career fairs, newspaper want ads, and employment websites. Additionally, professional associations, such as the American Association of Pharmaceutical Scientists and the American Society for Pharmacology and Experimental Therapeutics, provide job listings at their websites. See For More Information for a list of organizations. Those interested in positions with the federal government should visit the U.S. Office of Personnel Management's website, www.usajobs.opm.gov.

ADVANCEMENT

Medical scientists advance by receiving higher pay, by working on research projects that are more prestigious or offer larger budgets, by taking on managerial duties, or by becoming college professors and receiving tenure.

EARNINGS

Median annual salaries for medical scientists were $74,590 in 2009, according to the U.S. Department of Labor (USDL). Salaries ranged from less than $41,320 to $138,840 or more. The USDL reports the following mean annual earnings for medical scientists by employer: management, scientific, and technical consulting services, $113,250; federal government, $111,810; medical and diagnostic laboratories, $107,490; management of companies and enterprises, $104,400; scientific research and development services, $92,130; pharmaceutical and medicine manufacturing, $91,720; general medical and surgical hospitals, $76,520; and colleges, universities, and professional schools, $65,040. Salaries for epidemiologists ranged from less than $40,860 to $92,610 or more in 2009.

Medical scientists usually receive benefits such as health and life insurance, vacation days, sick leave, and a savings and pension plan. Self-employed scientists must provide their own benefits.

EMPLOYMENT OUTLOOK

Employment for medical scientists-except epidemiologists is expected to grow much faster than the average for all careers through 2018, according to the U.S. Department of Labor. Employment for epidemiologists is expected to grow faster than the average during this same time span. The growth of the biotechnology industry has fueled employment opportunities for medical scientists and will continue to do so in the next decade. Other factors that are influencing the strong employment outlook are the increasing number of people age 65 and older, which is creating demand for more drugs and therapies; the expansion in research related to illnesses such as cancer and avian flu, as well as treatment issues such as antibiotic resistance; and the increasing ease of travel and the growing world population, which will increase the chances of epidemics and pandemics and other global health outbreaks. Medical scientists who have both a Ph.D. and an M.D. will experience the best job prospects.

FOR MORE INFORMATION

For information on education and careers, contact the following organizations

American Association of Pharmaceutical Scientists
2107 Wilson Boulevard, Suite 700
Arlington, VA 22201-3046
www.aapspharmaceutica.com

American Society for Pharmacology and Experimental Therapeutics
9650 Rockville Pike
Bethesda, MD 20814-3995
www.aspet.org

continued on page 107

continued from page 106

For information on careers, contact
American Society for Microbiology
1752 N Street, NW
Washington, DC 20036-2904
202-737-3600
www.asm.org

For information about the benefits of
biotechnology research, visit the BIO
website.
**Biotechnology Industry
Organization (BIO)**
1201 Maryland Avenue, SW, Suite 900
Washington, DC 20024-6129
202-962-9200
info@bio.org
www.bio.org

For information on biotechnology
careers and industry facts, visit the
institute's website.
Biotechnology Institute
2000 North 14th Street, Suite 700
Arlington, VA 22201-2500
703-248-8681
info@biotechinstitute.org
www.biotechinstitute.org

The federation consists of 23 scientific societies with more than 100,000
researcher-members throughout the
world. Visit its website for more
information.
**Federation of American Societies
for Experimental Biology**
9650 Rockville Pike
Bethesda, MD 20814-3999
301-634-7000
info@faseb.org
www.faseb.org

For detailed information about biotechnology, visit the center's website.
**National Center
for Biotechnology Information**
National Library of Medicine
Building 38A
Bethesda, MD 20894
info@ncbi.nlm.nih.gov
www.ncbi.nlm.nih.gov

For information on pharmaceutical
and biotechnology research, contact
**Pharmaceutical Research and
Manufacturers of America**
950 F Street, NW, Suite 300
Washington, DC 20004-1440
202-835-3400
www.phrma.org

For information on epidemiology,
contact the following organizations
and government agencies
**Association for Professionals in
Infection Control and Epidemiology**
1275 K Street, NW, Suite 1000
Washington, DC 20005-4006
202-789-1890
apicinfo@apic.org
www.apic.org

**Centers for Disease
Control and Prevention**
1600 Clifton Road, NE
Atlanta, GA 30333-4018
800-232-4636
cdcinfo@cdc.gov
www.cdc.gov/phtrain/epidemiology.html

**Council of State and
Territorial Epidemiologists**
2872 Woodstock Boulevard, Suite 303
Atlanta, GA 30341-4015
770-458-3811
www.cste.org/dnn

Epidemic Intelligence Service
Centers for Disease Control and
Prevention
1600 Clifton Road, NE, Mailstop E-92
Atlanta, GA 30333-4018
404-498-6110
EIS@cdc.gov
www.cdc.gov/eis/index.html

**Infectious Diseases
Society of America**
1300 Wilson Boulevard, Suite 300
Arlington, VA 22209-2332
info@idsociety.org
www.idsociety.org

MENTAL HEALTH COUNSELORS

OVERVIEW

Mental health counselors work with individuals, families, and groups to identify and treat mental and emotional disorders and promote mental health. They help clients address issues such as depression, stress, anxiety, suicidal impulses, low self-esteem, addiction and substance abuse, trauma, and grief. In order to treat the individual, they may collaborate with other mental health specialists and professionals, such as psychiatrists, psychologists, clinical social workers, and school counselors. A minimum of a master's degree in counseling is required to work in the field. There are approximately 113,300 mental health counselors employed in the United States. Employment for mental health counselors is expected to grow much faster than the average for all careers through 2018.

FAST FACTS

High School Subjects
English
Psychology
Sociology

Personal Skills
Active listening
Communication
Helping

Minimum Education Level
Master's degree

Salary Range
$24,000 to $38,000 to $64,000+

Employment Outlook
Much faster than the average

O*NET-SOC
21-1011.00, 21-1014.00

GOE
12.02.02

DOT
045

NOC
4153

THE JOB

Many people suffer from anxiety or depression—whether due to stress at the workplace or school, a recent traumatic experience, grief from a death in the family, or low self-esteem resulting from divorce or job loss. Others suffer from drug addiction or alcohol abuse. Those with serious emotional impairments may even have suicidal tendencies. People turn to mental health counselors to help them deal with their various issues and bring them back to mental health.

Mental health counselors encourage patients to express their feelings—sadness, despair, or anger or discuss situations that occurred in their school or workplace, at home, in the military, or in other settings that left them particularly anxious or overwhelmed. Through these counseling sessions, counselors are able to help patients work through their feelings and establish strategies to overcome future episodes. Weekly sessions are typical, though patients, or counselors, may request more frequent sessions as needed.

When working with a new patient, mental health counselors first conduct a patient assessment. They ask the patient questions regarding physical health as well as for any other information that may give them a better picture of his or her mental state. When working with teens or young children, mental health counselors may first meet with the parents or guardians. They maintain detailed records and notes for each patient, which are confidential. During each session, mental health counselors actively listen to the patient, giving full attention to points being made and asking questions or giving prompts only when necessary. Counseling sessions occur one to one, though at times it is necessary to hold group sessions, such as in cases dealing with divorce, in which case entire families may be present. If patients suffer from alcohol or drug dependence, mental health counselors often include family members or close friends in some sessions to identify trigger situations associated with this dependency.

Mental health counselors also collect information through interviews, observation, and testing. They also collaborate with other professionals who are treating or interacting with the patient, such as physicians, nurses, teachers, and social workers. Using this information, they develop and implement a treatment plan for the patient. During the course of the treatment plan and counseling session, mental health counselors often meet with the patient's team of health professionals, as well as with the patient's family members and friends, to keep them abreast of the patient's progress. Some family members may even seek the counselor's advice on how to best deal with the patient's actions and recovery process.

Mental health counselors are excellent listeners. Instead of judging their patients' feelings or actions, counselors help patients by planning, organizing, and leading counseling programs. They teach patients alternative ways to deal with anger or resentment; for example, using behavioral therapy. They may use psychoanalysis to help patients understand their feelings of angst or despair. Mental health counselors also use different methods when working with young children, such as play therapy or art therapy, to learn the children's true emotions or fears.

As the patient improves, mental health counselors will begin to shift their sessions toward a plan for maintaining optimum mental health after therapy. This could include follow-up visits or phone calls for a period of time.

Counseling sessions take place in a quiet and private area, with only the patient and mental health counselor present. Mental health counselors take care to maintain a serene environment by providing a counseling area that is softly lit with comfortable couches or face-to-face seating.

Mental health counselors must stay up to date regarding new techniques, studies, or research through continuing-education courses, by attending seminars, or by reading professional literature. Some counselors serve their communities by running workshops to promote mental health issues and programs to prevent substance abuse.

Depending on their specialty, mental health counselors can work in many different environments such as classrooms, health centers, hospitals, day treatment programs, and governmental agencies. Some treat patients in private practice.

Mental health counselors work a standard 40-hour week, though many reserve evening or weekend hours to accommodate patients' work or school schedules. Since emergencies arise at all hours of the day or night, mental health counselors must be on call at all times. Those employed in a group setting may take turns being on call for patient emergencies, either via a pager or phone or through an answering service. Mental health counselors in private practice may take emergency calls through similar measures, as well as taking call turns with other colleagues.

Patient interaction accounts for a large part of a mental health counselor's day—either during counseling sessions or during assessments. Many times, mental health counselors are faced with helping patients who are severely agitated, depressed, or angry. It's important when working with such patients for mental health counselors to stay calm and professional, no matter the situation.

Oftentimes, patients have more than one health care professionals assigned to their care. Mental health counselors may be required to work with nurses, physicians, or social workers to collectively plan the best care and therapy program for the patient. They monitor the patient's prescribed medications and keep in touch with physicians regarding any problems. They many also confer with the patient's family and friends regarding any potential situations or problems at home or in the workplace.

Mental health counselors also supervise other counselors, assistants, or social service staff members. Additional duties depend upon where the mental health counselor is employed—whether at a hospital or agency or self-employed in a private practice. Those in private practice have additional administrative duties such as office maintenance, insurance paperwork, marketing, and billing. A counselor may also hire office assistants to handle these responsibilities.

Did You Know?

Approximately 20 percent of American youth suffer some type of mental disorder to the degree that it affects their ability to function, according to a survey by the National Institute of Mental Health (NIMH) published in the *Journal of the American Academy of Child and Adolescent Psychiatry*. In addition, "11 percent reported being severely impaired by a mood disorder (e.g., depression or bipolar disorder); 10 percent reported being severely impaired by a behavior disorder such as attention deficit hyperactivity disorder or conduct disorder; and 8 percent reported being severely impaired by at least one type of anxiety disorder."

Researchers at the NIMH analyzed data from the National Comorbidity Study-Adolescent Supplement, a national, face-to-face survey of more than 10,000 teens ages 13 to 18.

REQUIREMENTS

HIGH SCHOOL

In high school, take courses in psychology, English, and speech. Take as many science classes as possible, including biology, chemistry, and anatomy and physiology.

POSTSECONDARY TRAINING

You will need a master's degree to become a licensed mental health counselor, which is typically one of the job requirements set by employers. The Council for Accreditation of Counseling and Related Educational Programs accredits counseling programs. Visit its website, www.cacrep.org, for a list of programs.

CERTIFICATION AND LICENSING

Certification and licensing requirements vary greatly based on whether the counselor works for a private or public employer and by state law (although most states have laws requiring counselors to have some form of licensure). Contact the American Mental Health Counselors Association for information about certification and licensing requirements.

Some counselors choose to become certified by the National Board for Certified Counselors (NBCC, www.nbcc.org). This organization awards a general practice credential of national certified counselor. According to the U.S. Department of Labor, "this national certification is voluntary and is distinct from state licensing. However, in some states, those who pass the national exam are exempt from taking a state certification exam." The NBCC also offers specialty certifications in clinical mental health, addiction, and school counseling.

OTHER REQUIREMENTS

Key traits of mental health counselors include empathy, a strong desire to help others, good listening skills, the ability to communicate well both orally and in writing, strong ethics, the ability to work independently or as part of a team, and physical and mental energy to deal with sometimes stressful and demanding situations (as well as heartbreaking stories).

EXPLORING

There are many ways to learn more about a career as a mental health counselor. You can read books and journals (such as the *Journal of Mental Health Counseling,* www.amhca.org/news/journal.aspx) about the field, visit the websites of college counseling programs to learn about typical classes and possible career paths, and ask your teacher or school counselor to arrange an information interview with a mental health counselor. Professional associations can also provide information about the field. The American Mental Health Counselors Association provides information on careers at its website, www.amhca.org. You should also try to land a part-time job in the office of a mental health counselor. This will give you a chance to interact with counselors and see if the career is a good fit for your interests and abilities.

EMPLOYERS

There are approximately 113,300 mental health counselors employed in the United States. They work for managed behavioral health care organizations, substance abuse treatment centers, community agencies, hospitals, employee assistance programs, and other organizations and government agencies that provide mental health services. Additionally, some mental health counselors work in private practice or teach counseling at colleges and universities.

GETTING A JOB

Many mental health counselors obtain their first jobs as a result of contacts made through college internships or networking events. Others seek assistance in obtaining job leads from college career services offices, newspaper want ads, and employment websites. Additionally, professional associations, such as the American Counseling Association (ACA), provide job listings at their websites. The ACA also provides helpful articles on writing résumés, acing job interviews, and other career-oriented topics. See For More Information for contact information for the ACA and other organizations. Those interested in positions with the federal government should visit the U.S. Office of Personnel Management's website, www.usajobs.opm.gov.

ADVANCEMENT

Salaried mental health counselors advance by receiving increases in pay and managerial duties. Self-employed counselors advance by developing a strong reputation in their community and attracting more clients. Some counselors become college professors and/or write textbooks about mental health counseling.

EARNINGS

Salaries for mental health counselors vary by type of employer, geographic region, and the worker's experience, education, and skill level. Median annual salaries for mental health counselors were $38,010 in 2009, according to the U.S. Department of Labor (USDL). Salaries ranged from less than $24,230 to $64,610 or more. The USDL reports the following mean annual earnings for mental health counselors by employer: home health care services, $54,090; elementary and secondary schools, $57,120; local government, $49,630; offices of other health practitioners, $45,610; outpatient care centers, $41,210; individual and family services, $39,710; and residential mental retardation, mental health, and substance abuse facilities, $33,020.

Mental health counselors usually receive benefits such as health and life insurance, vacation days, sick leave, and a savings and pension plan. Self-employed workers must provide their own benefits.

EMPLOYMENT OUTLOOK

Employment for mental health counselors is expected to grow much faster than the average for all careers through 2018, according to the U.S. Department of Labor. There will be more jobs available (especially in rural areas) than there are people graduating with degrees in counseling. Mental health counselors will enjoy good employment prospects because there is growing demand for mental health services and increasing insurance reimbursements for the services of counselors (which are causing them to be sought after by health care providers as cost-effective alternatives to psychiatrists and psychologists).

FOR MORE INFORMATION

For information on suicide prevention, contact
American Association of Suicidology
5221 Wisconsin Avenue, NW
Washington, DC 20015-2032
202-237-2280 |
www.suicidology.org

For information on certification and the job search, contact
American Counseling Association
5999 Stevenson Avenue
Alexandria, VA 22304-3304
800-347-6647
www.counseling.org

For information on mental health counseling, contact
American Mental Health Counselors Association
801 North Fairfax Street, Suite 304
Alexandria, VA 22314-1775
800-326-2642
www.amhca.org

For information on psychotherapy, contact
American Psychotherapy Association
2750 East Sunshine Street
Springfield, MO 65804-2047
800-205-9165
www.americanpsychotherapy.com

For information on accredited programs, contact
Council for Accreditation of Counseling and Related Educational Programs
American Counseling Association
1001 North Fairfax Street, Suite 510
Alexandria, VA 22314-1587
703-535-5990
www.cacrep.org

For information about mental health issues, contact the following organizations
Mental Health America
2000 North Beauregard Street, 6th Floor
Alexandria, VA 22311
800-969-6642
www.nmha.org

National Institute of Mental Health
National Institutes of Health
Science Writing, Press, and Dissemination Branch
6001 Executive Boulevard, Room 8184, MSC 9663
Bethesda, MD 20892-9663
nimhinfo@nih.gov
www.nimh.nih.gov

For information on certification, contact
National Board for Certified Counselors
3 Terrace Way, Suite D
Greensboro, NC 27403-3660
336-547-0607
nbcc@nbcc.org
www.nbcc.org

NURSING AIDES

OVERVIEW

Nursing aides provide care to patients in hospitals, nursing homes, mental health facilities, patients' homes, and other health care settings. They perform routine tasks such as feeding, bathing, dressing, or transporting patients—all under the supervision of nurses or other medical staff. A minimum of a high school diploma is required to work as a nursing aide. Nearly 1.5 million nursing aides are employed in the United States. Employment is expected to be excellent for nursing aides through 2018. Nursing aides are also known as *nursing assistants, nurse aides, direct care workers, certified nursing assistants, care assistants, hospice assistants, patient care assistants, restorative aides, geriatric aides, orderlies,* and *hospital attendants.*

FAST FACTS

High School Subjects
Biology
Health

Personal Skills
Following instructions
Helping

Minimum Education Level
High school diploma

Salary Range
$17,000 to $24,000 to $33,000+

Employment Outlook
Faster than the average

O*NET-SOC
31-1012.00

GOE
14.07.01

DOT
354

NOC
3413

THE JOB

The main duty of nursing aides is patient care. They prepare patients for the day by bathing, grooming, and dressing them. If the patient is unable to stand unassisted, oftentimes nursing aides may need to secure the patient by using specially designed shower seats or bathtub seats before completing the task. Bedridden patients are given a bed bath and changed into fresh hospital gowns. Once patients are dressed, nursing aides help them, depending on their condition, into wheelchairs or wheeled gurneys, or situated into dayrooms or other activity centers. Some patients are transported for therapies, treatments, or appointments.

Nursing aides must be careful when assisting patients out of beds and into wheelchairs. Too quick a movement or not using proper momentum can cause physical harm to the nursing aide as well as the patient. Devices such as the Hoyer lift or other hydraulic mechanisms are helpful in easily and safely transferring obese or physically challenged patients.

Mealtimes are busy for nursing aides. They help distribute meal trays and help patients eat, if necessary. Assistance can range from opening food wrappers and bottle caps, to cutting meat into small pieces, to mixing food and feeding the patient by hand. Nursing aides may test diabetics for their blood sugar in the morning to make sure levels are safe. Nursing aides are also responsible for picking up food trays after each meal and helping patients who need an extra napkin or help washing their hands.

Toilet assistance is another duty of nursing aides. Some patients may call for help in transferring to the bathroom toilet or portable toilet chair, while others prefer to use the bedpan or urinal. Nursing aides clean patients who are incontinent, changing them into fresh clothing.

Nursing aides may take patients' vital signs (such as temperature, pulse, and blood pressure), documenting each reading on the patients' charts or in an electronic database. Some nursing aides are specially trained to assist in exercises as designed by physical and occupational therapists. They may also be asked to participate alongside patients in social activities such as holiday celebrations, birthdays, or other occasions.

Nursing aides also keep track of supplies such as gloves, linens, towels, and other patient care items. They change linens and tidy up each patient's room and bathroom area. Nursing aides may also provide fresh ice water and juice or toiletry items, as requested. Other duties of nursing aides include helping patients take daily walks, turning bedridden patients regularly, and moving equipment and supplies in and out of patients' rooms.

If a patient under their care dies, nursing aides are responsible for cleaning the patient, gathering his or her personal possessions, and preparing the patient for transportation to the morgue. When a room is vacated, nursing aides clean and disinfect the area before a new patient is brought in.

Nursing aides monitor patients' physical, mental, and emotional status and inform the nursing staff of any changes. In addition to their daily patient care duties, nursing aides may receive other tasks or assignments from their supervising nurse or special requests from patients. Some duties differ according to the nursing aide's work shift. For example, day shift assignments revolve around getting patients ready for their daily activities and eating breakfast and lunch; night shift assignments revolve around eating dinner and preparing patients for bed.

Full-time nursing aides usually work eight-hour shifts, 40 hours a week. Some shifts are scheduled during the evenings, weekends, and holidays.

The work is physically demanding, as nursing aides are often standing, stooping, walking, or lifting heavy patients. They also risk bodily injury, especially to the back, when lifting and transferring patients from one location to another. It's important for nursing aides to understand and practice the proper procedures for lifting and transferring patients in order to avoid injuries. Nursing aides also are at risk of contracting illnesses (such as HIV or hepatitis) from their patients; they wear protective gloves and masks to reduce this risk.

There are many unpleasant tasks involved in work as a nursing aide, including emptying bedpans, changing soiled linens, and cleaning patients when they are incontinent. At times, nursing aides may work with patients who are depressed, angry, or confused. Some patients may even become violent. Despite these negatives, most nursing aides enjoy their jobs. They find it rewarding to help others. Many times, nursing aides are able to forge caring relationships with their patients, especially those requiring daily, long-term care.

REQUIREMENTS

HIGH SCHOOL

Recommended classes include health, psychology, biology, anatomy and physiology, computer science, English, and speech. Taking a foreign language such as Spanish will come in handy if you work in an area that has a large population that does not speak English as a first language. Some high schools offer formal training programs for prospective nursing aides.

POSTSECONDARY TRAINING

A minimum of a high school diploma is required to work as a nursing aide. Some nursing aides complete one- to two-year nurse aide programs at community colleges. Other receive their training in formal employer-provided classroom instruction or through on-the-job training. Classes cover topics such as anatomy and physiology, infection control, body mechanics, nutrition, communication skills, personal-care skills, and medical ethics. Students often also complete an internship or clinical experience as part of their studies.

CERTIFICATION AND LICENSING

Nursing aides who work in nursing care facilities must be certified. Aides that satisfactorily complete a state-approved training program of at least 75 hours and pass a competency evaluation can use the designation, certified nurse assistant. Some states have additional requirements. Contact your state's board of professional regulation for information on requirements in your state.

OTHER REQUIREMENTS

To be a successful nursing aide, you should have empathy and compassion for others. You should work well under pressure, be able to handle multiple—and sometimes repetitive—tasks, be dependable, be good at following instructions, have patience, have excellent communication skills, and be able to work as a member of a team. You should also be in good physical and mental health and be able to pass state-mandated medical tests, as well as background checks administered by potential employers.

EXPLORING

There are many ways to learn more about a career as a nursing assistant. You can read books and magazines (such as *Caring* magazine, www.nahc.org) about the field, visit the websites of college nurse assistant programs to learn about typical classes and possible career paths, and ask

Learn More About It

Carter, Pamela J. *Lippincott's Textbook For Nursing Assistants: A Humanistic Approach to Caregiving.* 3rd ed. Philadelphia: Lippincott Williams & Wilkins, 2011.

LearningExpress LLC. *Nursing Assistant/Nurse Aide Exam.* 4th ed. New York: LearningExpress LLC, 2009.

Sorrentino, Sheila A., Leighann Remmert, and Bernie Gorek. *Mosby's Essentials for Nursing Assistants.* 4th ed. St. Louis: Mosby, 2009.

your teacher or school counselor to arrange an information interview with a nursing assistant. You should also try to land a part-time job as a nursing assistant. This will give you a chance to see if the career is a good fit for your interests and abilities.

EMPLOYERS

Nearly 1.5 million nursing aides are employed in the United States. Nursing care facilities employ about 41 percent of nursing aides, and 29 percent work in hospitals. Other employers include home health care agencies, government agencies, outpatient care centers, and residential care facilities.

GETTING A JOB

Many nursing assistants obtain their first jobs as a result of contacts made through college internships or practicums, career fairs, or networking events. Others seek assistance in obtaining job leads from college career services offices, newspaper want ads, and employment websites. Direct application to potential employers is another way nursing assistants obtain jobs. Those interested in positions with the federal government should visit the U.S. Office of Personnel Management's website, www.usajobs.opm.gov.

ADVANCEMENT

There are few advancement opportunities for nursing assistants unless they return to school to continue their education. Career paths for those who complete additional education include licensed practical nurse, registered nurse, and medical assistant.

EARNINGS

Salaries for nursing assistants vary by type of employer, geographic region, and the worker's experience, education, and skill level. Median annual salaries for nursing assistants were $24,040 in 2009, according to the U.S. Department of Labor (USDL). Salaries ranged from less than $17,510 to

$33,970 or more. The USDL reports the following mean annual earnings for nursing assistants by employer: local government, $27,140; general medical and surgical hospitals, $26,540; nursing care facilities, $24,080; community care facilities for the elderly, $23,320; and home health care services, $23,070.

Full-time nursing assistants usually receive benefits such as health and life insurance, vacation days, sick leave, and a savings and pension plan. Part-time workers must provide their own benefits. Approximately 24 percent of nursing aides work part time.

EMPLOYMENT OUTLOOK

Employment is expected to be excellent for nursing aides through 2018, according to the U.S. Department of Labor. In fact, approximately 276,000 new jobs are expected to be available from 2008 to 2018. Steady increases in the elderly population, whose members typically require more medical care than people in other age demographics, are creating demand for nursing aides. In addition, technological advances are allowing physicians to save more people from diseases and injuries that would have been fatal in the past—creating a need for qualified caregivers for these individuals. Nursing and residential care facilities—especially community care facilities for the elderly—will offer the best employment prospects in coming years.

There is high turnover in the field because it is mentally and physically demanding to work as a nursing aide, there are few advancement opportunities for those who do not receive additional education, and the pay is low. Many people work as nursing aides while attending college programs to prepare for careers in other health care fields such as nursing or physician assisting.

OCCUPATIONAL THERAPISTS

OVERVIEW

Occupational therapists work with patients who are suffering from mentally, physically, developmentally, or emotionally disabling conditions. They help patients improve their ability to perform daily-living and work-related tasks. Using exercises or programs to increase strength, visual acuity, or performance, occupational therapists teach patients how to live independently and have productive lives. A minimum of a master's degree in occupational therapy is required to enter the field. Approximately 104,500 occupational therapists are employed in the United States. Employment in the field is expected to grow much faster than the average for all careers through 2018.

FAST FACTS

High School Subjects
Biology
Health

Personal Skills
Helping
Problem solving

Minimum Education Level
Master's degree

Salary Range
$45,000 to $69,000 to $100,000+

Employment Outlook
Much faster than the average

O*NET-SOC
29-1122.00

GOE
14.06.01

DOT
076

NOC
3143

THE JOB

People sometimes are physically or mentally limited due to the effects of illness, injury, age, or a physical or psychological condition. These limitations can affect the way they live, work, play, and even learn. People often turn to occupational therapists to help them cope and adjust their activities in a way that makes them more productive, mobile, and independent.

Occupational therapists use games, activities, exercises, and various equipment and tools to improve a patient's basic motor functions and his or her basic reasoning skills. Activities or adaptations may also be designed to compensate for permanent loss of function. Occupational therapists work with patients with a wide range of conditions—from those recuperating from illness or accident, to those with developmental issues—and ages, from infants to senior citizens. While many patients undergo a combination of physical and occupational therapy programs, there is a big difference between the two disciplines. Physical therapy works to restore movement and mobility, while occupational therapy focuses on fine motor skills to restore function.

When working with a new patient, occupational therapists must first assess the patient's needs in all areas—home, work, and recreation. Occupational therapists identify problem areas or activities in their client's home or workplace, and they work to remove the barriers or help the patient make necessary adaptations. For example, when working with a patient who has severe arthritis, occupational therapists may create adaptive equipment for, say, cooking or gardening, to make those particular tasks easier and more productive. Occupational therapists may introduce patients to ergonomic cooking tools, gardening equipment, or other assistive devices to improve mobility and dexterity in these areas.

Top Emerging Practice Areas

✔ Addressing the psychosocial needs of children and youth

✔ Design and accessibility consulting and home modification

✔ Driver rehabilitation and training

✔ Ergonomics consulting

✔ Health and wellness consulting

✔ Low vision services

✔ Private practice community health services

✔ Technology and assistive device development and consulting

✔ Ticket to Work and Work Incentives Improvement Act services

✔ Welfare-to-work services

Source: American Occupational Therapy Association

Once problem areas are identified, occupational therapists assist the patient to develop, maintain, or, in some cases, relearn skills to a more satisfactory level of living and play. Some occupational therapists practice general therapy, meaning they treat people of all ages and conditions. However, most occupational therapists specialize in a particular area, such as pediatrics, gerontology, rehabilitation, or psychiatry.

Pediatric occupational therapists work with infants, children, and adolescents with a variety of conditions, including developmental delays; delays in gross, fine, motor, or visual skills; autistic-spectrum delays; and even children with adoption-related concerns. In addition, pediatric occupational therapists work with age-appropriate patients needing help due to illness, disease, or injuries. Early-intervention therapy is important for infants and toddlers who may be at risk for developmental delays as identified by their parents, pediatrician, or teacher.

Tools and equipment, many of which are play based, are often tailored to fit the age, size, and attention span of children. Some sessions may be one on one, while others are held in a group setting. Therapists may have children play with modeling clay, hammer sets, or other toys to stimulate fine motor skills. They teach children different grasps to help them better hold a pencil or other writing implement. Occupational therapists use therapeutic listening techniques to help children improve their attention spans, behavior, and cognitive processing, which in turn will help them perform better in school. Other therapies help children develop their social skills or teach them skills used for dressing and grooming.

As people age, many find it harder to perform many activities and tasks due to increasing sensory impairment and conditions common with older populations, such as arthritis or Alzheimer's disease. Occupational therapy for gerontology greatly helps the elderly lead more independent and active lives. *Gerontological occupational therapists* may give patients exercises to compensate for difficult movements. Tools such as a bilateral sander—a box with handles on either side—require patients to move the handles backwards and forwards, or side to side, which improves strength and range of motion. Attaching and detaching Velcro blocks can also improve strength and dexterity, both of which are needed for many of the patient's activities of daily living. Cognitive games such as cards, peg boards, or other activities can improve a patient's memory and critical-thinking skills. Other tools and techniques are used to improve patients' cooking, grooming, or dressing skills, as well as other activities that are important to the patients' lives and well-being.

After assessing the patient's home, an occupational therapist may suggest adaptive aides such as safety bars or handles for the bathtub, shower, or toilet area to prevent accidents. They also suggest walking aids or techniques to improve speed and prevent injuries. Some therapists specially trained in driver rehabilitation can teach elderly patients skills to be better and safer drivers.

Rehabilitation is another occupational therapy specialty. Patients recovering from injury or conditions such as a stroke or heart attack often need therapy to help them assimilate back into their everyday lives. For example, stroke patients with short-term memory loss may be taught to make lists or other reminder cues to help in recall. Occupational therapists may use computer games to help patients improve their sequencing, coordination, and problem-solving skills. Exercises done with rubber balls, bands, and other tools can also be implemented to help improve strength and dexterity. Patients suffering from vision loss can be taught techniques to make better use of their remaining vision or can be trained with adaptive equipment such as audio recordings, talking devices, computer technology, or special writing materials. Occupational therapists also help patients use adaptive equipment such as wheelchairs or orthotics. Sometimes, occupational therapists design special tools to better fit a patient's condition, needs, or environment including grasping claws to reach items, computer-aided equipment for communication, or other aids to facilitate dressing, eating, grooming, and other daily tasks.

Psychiatric occupational therapists help patients with acute mental health conditions or learning disabilities. Activities, which are geared to improve skills such as time management and socialization, give patients the confidence to live independently or take part in social activities. Occupational therapists also work with patients suffering from alcoholism, drug addiction, depression, eating disorders, or stress-related conditions. They can help patients improve their skills to do everyday tasks such as shopping, cooking, cleaning, using public transportation, or even holding a job.

Occupational therapists also have administrative duties. After each session, they track and chart a patient's progress. They often consult with physicians, nurses, social workers, and other health care professionals regarding a patient's condition or treatment plan. Some occupational therapists supervise occupational therapy assistants, medical assistants, or volunteers.

Approximately 31 percent of occupational therapists employed in the United States work part-time, with some working for more than one employer at various times. Full-time therapists work about 40 hours a week, with some evening and weekend hours scheduled. Occupational therapists can expect to work indoors in large, spacious, well-lit workrooms. Some work is done outdoors, especially when conducting activities such as gardening, games, exercises, or perhaps practice visits to various stores. At times, occupational therapists make follow-up visits to patients' homes, schools, or workplaces to determine their rate of progress.

This career can be demanding and tiring; occupational therapists spend much of their day on their feet or walking from activity to activity. They also run the risk of injury—especially to their back—when supporting, lifting, or shifting patients, or when moving heavy equipment.

REQUIREMENTS

HIGH SCHOOL

Take courses in anatomy and physiology, biology, chemistry, health, physics, psychology, art, computer science, and the social sciences.

POSTSECONDARY TRAINING

There are no baccalaureate-level occupational therapy programs. Aspiring occupational therapists typically earn undergraduate degrees in anatomy, anthropology, biology, kinesiology, liberal arts, psychology, or sociology.

You will need a minimum of a master's degree in occupational therapy to work in the field. Combined bachelor's/master's degree programs are available for those who have not earned a bachelor's degree before entry into an occupational therapy educational program. Visit the American Occupational Therapy Association's website, www.aota.org/Students/Schools.aspx, for a list of approximately 150 occupational therapy programs that are accredited by the Association.

Typical classes include Introduction to Occupational Sciences and Occupational Therapy, Kinesiology for the Occupational Therapist, Theoretical Foundations of Occupational Therapy, Technologies in

Occupational Therapy, Occupations of Infants and Children, Applied Neuroscience for Occupational Therapy, Research and Occupational Therapy, Occupations of Adolescents and Young Adults, Pathophysiology: Impact of Conditions on Occupation, Occupations of Adults and Older Adults, and Professional Trends and Issues in Occupational Therapy. In addition to classes, students participate in at least 24 hours of fieldwork, where they work with patients under the supervision of experienced occupational therapists.

CERTIFICATION AND LICENSING

National certification is available from the National Board for Certification in Occupational Therapy (NBCOT). Certification is required as one criterion of becoming licensed. To become certified, you must graduate from an accredited occupational therapy program, complete the clinical practice period, and pass a written test. Those who meet these requirements are awarded the designation, occupational therapist, registered. In addition, the NBCOT offers several specialty certifications, including board certification in gerontology, mental health, pediatrics, and physical rehabilitation, as well as specialty certification in driving and community mobility; environmental modification; feeding, eating, and swallowing; and low vision.

All states and the District of Columbia require occupational therapists to be licensed or meet other forms of professional regulation. To become licensed, you must graduate from an accredited occupational therapy program, and then take and pass the NBCOT certification exam. In some states, you must meet additional requirements, such as passing an exam that measures your knowledge of state statutes and regulations.

OTHER REQUIREMENTS

The ability to communicate well is important for occupational therapists, who teach, instruct, and motivate their patients when working with them one on one. In addition, they frequently write reports detailing their treatment plans for patients and document their progress. A successful occupational therapist will remain emotionally calm and stable when dealing with sometimes stressed, angry, or uncooperative patients. Other important traits for occupational therapists include patience, imagination, creativity, and good problem-solving skills.

EXPLORING

Does the career of occupational therapist sound interesting? If so, there are many ways to learn more about this career. You can read books and journals (such as *OT Practice,* www.aota.org/Pubs/OTP.aspx) about the field, visit the websites of college occupational therapy programs to learn about typical classes and possible career paths, and ask your teacher or school counselor to arrange an information interview with an occupational therapist. Professional associations can also provide information about the field. The American Occupational Therapy Association provides a lot of helpful information on education and careers at its website, www.aota.org/Students/Prospective.aspx. You should also try to land a part-time job in the office of an occupational therapist. This will give you a chance to interact with therapists and assistants and see if the career is a good fit for your interests and abilities.

EMPLOYERS

Approximately 104,500 occupational therapists are employed in the United States. Occupational therapists are employed by hospitals; nursing homes; intermediate-care facilities; public and private schools; mental-health centers; rehabilitation hospitals; home health agencies; group homes; individual and family services; community care facilities for the elderly; offices of physicians and other health care practitioners; government agencies; and outpatient clinics. A small number of occupational therapists work in private practice.

GETTING A JOB

Many occupational therapists obtain their first jobs as a result of contacts made through college internships, career fairs, or networking events. Others seek assistance in obtaining job leads from college career services offices, newspaper want ads, and employment websites. Additionally, the American Occupational Therapy Association provides job listings at its website, www.otjoblink.org. Those interested in positions with the federal government should visit the U.S. Office of Personnel Management's website, www.usajobs.opm.gov.

ADVANCEMENT

Occupational therapists advance by receiving increases in salary and managerial duties. Others become sought-after specialists in gerontology, mental health, pediatrics, physical rehabilitation, or other areas. Occupational therapists also work as professors at colleges and universities.

EARNINGS

Salaries for occupational therapists vary by type of employer, geographic region, and the worker's experience, education, and skill level. Median annual salaries for occupational therapists were $69,630 in 2009, according to the U.S. Department of Labor (USDL). Salaries ranged from less than $45,340 to $100,430 or more. The USDL reports the following mean annual earnings for occupational therapists by employer: home health care services, $81,360; nursing care facilities, $75,710; offices of other health care practitioners, $72,970; general medical and surgical hospitals, $71,300; and elementary and secondary schools, $63,190.

Employers offer a variety of benefits, including the following: medical, dental, and life insurance; paid holidays, vacations, and sick and personal days; 401(k) plans; profit-sharing plans; retirement and pension plans; and educational-assistance programs. Self-employed therapists must provide their own benefits.

EMPLOYMENT OUTLOOK

An increase in the number of people who have disabilities or who have limited function, growth in the number of individuals age 65 and over (who often have a higher incidence of illness and disability), and advances in medical technology and therapy techniques will create strong opportunities for occupational therapy professionals through 2018, according to the U.S. Department of Labor (USDL). In fact, the USDL predicts that employment for occupational therapists will increase much faster than the average for all occupations during this time span, with job opportunities "good for licensed occupational therapists in all settings, particularly in acute hospital, rehabilitation, and orthopedic settings because the elderly receive most of their treatment in these settings." The American Occupational Therapy Association reports that opportunities should be good in early-intervention programs and in schools for children with disabilities served by the federal Individuals with Disabilities Education Act. Occupational therapists who have specialized knowledge in an area such as gerontology will have the best job prospects.

FOR MORE INFORMATION

Visit the association's Web site to learn more about accredited occupational therapy programs, career information, and news related to the field.
American Occupational Therapy Association
4720 Montgomery Lane
PO Box 31220
Bethesda, MD 20824-1220
301-652-2682
educate@aota.org
www.aota.org

For information on certification, contact
National Board for Certification in Occupational Therapy
12 South Summit Avenue, Suite 100
Gaithersburg, MD 20877-2090
301-990-7979
www.nbcot.org

Interview: Leslie Jackson

Leslie Jackson, M.Ed., OT, FAOTA is an occupational therapist who works as the family support project coordinator for Easter Seals, Inc. in Chicago, Illinois. She discussed her career with the editors of *Hot Health Care Careers*.

Q. How long have you worked in the field? What made you want to enter this career?

A. I have been an occupational therapist for 28 years and have always worked with children in a variety of settings, including school systems, inpatient rehab, early intervention and other home care, and private practice. I first learned about occupational therapy (OT) during a high school senior assignment and became intrigued, although I went into college as a music major. About halfway through my freshman year, I decided to change my major to Pre-OT and haven't looked back since. I currently work for Easter Seals, Inc., the Easter Seals headquarters office. Easter Seals is one of the largest providers of services and support for children and adults with disabilities in the country (see our website, www. easterseals.com, for more information). I coordinate a federally funded training project that provides training and information for families of children with disabilities and advocates on available sources of support and how to access them.

Q.   What is one thing that young people may not know about a career in occupational therapy?

A.   They might not even know what occupational therapy—or what we affectionately call OT—is. The field seems to be a well-kept secret, even with efforts to tell folks about who we are and what we do. Most of the folks that I talk to have "heard about" physical therapy or nursing, or being a lawyer or a slew of other professions, but not OT unless they know someone with a disability or have had direct contact with a therapist.

Q.   What are the most important personal and professional qualities for occupational therapists?

A.   You have to like working with people, first and foremost, because therapists spend a great deal of time getting to know their clients, what's important to them and how to help them do those everyday activities. Creativity and flexibility are also important because we are often challenged to find solutions that work for our clients; some solutions may or may not be a good fit or may not have worked before. Sometimes, these solutions will work for many clients, and sometimes we have to fashion some very specific ones for a particular client. Another personal trait is to be inquisitive, to want to explore and investigate all options in order to find the "just right" solution for our clients.

Q.   What are some of the pros and cons of your job?

A.   All jobs/professions have pros and cons. For me, the pros far outweigh the cons. I love working with the children and figuring out how to best help them and their families do the things that are important to them; to learn new ways of thinking about how to do what I do and find more effective ways to support the kids; and to be able to help other therapists become better at what they do.

Q.   What advice would you give to young people who are interested in becoming occupational therapists?

A.   I would tell them to spend time observing and talking to occupational therapists. Volunteer with people with disabilities in different settings. Ask themselves what kind of work they might want to do and what kind of people they want to work with. They might not know specific details, but do they like helping others, or do they want to "stay away from" people who are sick, disabled, not able to do for themselves? Do they think they might want to teach at a college or university or do research? Shadowing an occupational therapist and/or volunteering will let them see what is possible and whether this will be "good fit" for them and if they might have what it takes to make a great therapist.

Q. What is the employment outlook for occupational therapists? How is the field changing?

A. The employment outlook for occupational therapy is excellent. Occupational therapists are not limited in what they can do (e.g., educators, clinicians, administrators, researchers) or where they can work. They can work with children, adults, or both and can specialize in employment, pediatrics, geriatrics, hands, advocacy/lobbying, home health, burns, head injury, spinal cord injury, mental health, or technology, just to name some of the areas.

Interview: Melissa Winkle

Melissa Winkle, OTR/L is the owner of Dogwood Therapy Services, Inc. (www.dogwoodtherapy.com) in Albuquerque, New Mexico. She discussed her career with the editors of *Hot Health Care Careers*.

Q. How long have you worked in the field? What made you want to enter this career?

A. I graduated from the University of New Mexico in 2001. I became an occupational therapist after volunteering in a variety of therapeutic disciplines for four years. I watched the interactions of patients and clients with each discipline and loved the functionality of the scope of practice found in occupational therapy. When people work with occupational therapists, they are able to return to doing something that they have not been able to do for a period of time. Other clients learn how to do something that they have never been able to do before. Occupational therapists work with people of all ages and stages of life, who have encountered a disability due to birth, injury, illness, or aging. The goal is for them to become as independent as possible, or to regain their dignity and self-sufficiency. I was attracted to occupational therapy because it is the study of people and their roles, patterns, and habits. It encompasses extensive knowledge about the body and how it all works together so that people can establish or return to roles, patterns, and habits.

Q. What is one thing that young people may not know about a career in occupational therapy?

A. Occupational therapists are actually health care providers. The term "occupation" refers to what people do with their time—at different ages and stages of life, we all have different things that occupy our time. As children, our occupation is to play, grow, and learn. An occupational therapist may work with a child who has a disability in a hospital or clinical setting, at school, at home, or in the community. Their goals may be to learn how to use their fingers to manipulate buttons, zippers, and snaps; to learn play skills like climbing, to learn social skills, or to maintain standing balance to reach items on a table top; or to transition to new environments without having a behavioral outcome as a result of sensory processing issues. An occupational therapist (OT) might also work with a teen or an adult who suffered a spinal cord injury as the result of an accident. In this case therapies may take place in similar settings, and the client may even need skills to get back into the work setting. This person may need stretching, strengthening, and memory and other thinking skills. They may also need assistive technology such as splints or wheelchairs, or even voice-activated computers so they may resume normal activities or occupations. OTs may serve in the role of life coaching, as people begin making interesting life changes such as vocations, family status, returning from serving in the military, etc. Later in life, individuals may find themselves with diagnoses that are more common with aging. A person may have a stroke and lose the use of one side of his or her body and some thinking skills. In this case, an occupational therapist offers strategies for strength, balance, dressing, cooking, visual issues (loss of peripheral vision, etc), problem-solving strategies, etc.

Q. What are the most important personal and professional qualities for OTs?

A.   An occupational therapist must be able to work as an individual and as part of an interdisciplinary team alongside physicians, nurses, social workers, other therapy professionals, teachers, corrections officers, etc. It is critical that OTs be able to take perspective of others' situations, socioeconomic status, spiritual beliefs, and lifestyle. Disability happens to people from all walks of life and with little or no warning. OTs should be chameleons, and be able to blend into a person's home and family life, into a prison situation, into a daycare, or into a crowd on a bus. This is where people live and occupy their time. The best OTs are creative and flexible, and they spend a lot of time watching and listening.

Q. What are some of the pros and cons of your job?

A.   For me, the best part of occupational therapy is seeing people make progress, working in a variety of environments. I have worked in schools, homes, community centers, places of employment, clinics, hospitals, skilled nursing facilities, corrections facilities, and the greater community. I have worked with clients to drive, and to schedule transportation. I have taken clients on buses, taxis, trains, planes, and automobiles. I get to become part of people's lives; sometimes for a brief period, and others for much longer. Sometimes clients attend sessions with a friend or a family member—so our network can be rather large. I have been very fortunate to open a private practice and have a special interest in individuals with developmental disabilities and integrated services. Individuals are typically referred to us for our modalities of nature therapy, animal-assisted therapy, and assistance dogs as assistive-technology options. It is great to be working in the community, and later that afternoon, be working on research to prove the efficacy of our preferred modalities and methodologies.

Another exciting part of occupational therapy is that you are never done learning. There are always advances in health care, and there is always a lot to learn.

The most difficult part of occupational therapy is that services may be severely limited or there may be a waiting list for people to get funding for services. For example, it is not realistic for an individual who has received a traumatic brain injury and physical injuries to be able to return to daily routines after just 12 visits. In addition, the amount of documentation, which is different for each funding source, can feel overwhelming. There are evaluations, reports, intervention plans, support plans, progress reports, daily contact notes, and client working files to keep. Another downfall to occupational therapy is that people do not know what the profession really does.

Q. What advice would you give to young people who are interested in becoming occupational therapists?

A. Anyone interested in occupational therapy should volunteer in at least three different settings. Each will be totally different from the next. Each facility is as unique as the individuals who seek services. As I reflect on my career, I would advise young people to learn all you can in volunteer settings, in college, and on the job. But remember that there is no such thing as a textbook client.

Q. What is the employment outlook for occupational therapists? How is the field changing?

A. Occupational therapy is up and coming. While the field began its emergence in the 1700s, mainly in the psychiatric/psychosocial arena, the field has evolved into a strong holistic profession. OTs now have working knowledge and skills to facilitate self-help skills and independence in the triad of mind, body, and spirit in any environment that is meaningful to the individuals we serve.

Interview: Rondalyn Whitney

Rondalyn Whitney, MOT, OTR/L is an occupational therapist who works at the Center for Autism and Related Disorders at Kennedy Krieger Institute in Baltimore, Maryland as a researcher studying social skills for children with Autism Spectrum Disorder. She is the author of *Nonverbal Learning Disorder: Understanding and Coping with NLD and Asperger's-What Parents and Teachers Need to Know*. (Visit http://rondalynwhitney.com to learn more about her career and the field of occupational therapy.) Rondalyn discussed her career and the field of occupational therapy with the editors of *Hot Health Care Careers*.

Q. How long have you worked in the field? What made you want to enter this career?

A. I work at Kennedy Krieger Institute in the capacity of a research coordinator IV. As an occupational therapist (OT), I specialized with children with social relatedness problems, and I designed innovative occupational-based intervention programs for them both in private practice and school-based practice. I also worked as a consultant and trainer to school personnel, have published on my area of specialty, and have taught at the university level in occupational therapy programs. My background as an OT was critical in being hired for this amazing position.

I have been in the field of occupational therapy since 1993. I wanted to find a way to help patients deal with their disabilities and return to what was meaningful to them, to reestablish their connection to what brought them a sense of wholeness and a sense of well-being. I loved art, science, religious study, physiology, psychology, special education, neu-

rology, writing, working with people and solving problems, being creative, and work in medicine. I was told that was too eclectic, that I had
to narrow it down. I took an interest inventory at the career center during the junior year of my undergraduate program—it came out that I
should be a "window display designer" (no kidding) and that I should
find a vocation and create a lifestyle that would allow me to pursue my
many interests as 'hobbies.' I hadn't heard of occupational therapy, and
no one suggested it to me. I ended up with a B.A. in medical psychology
and a minor in interdisciplinary honors, which, when you look at the
courses I took, was consistent with the course work of an occupational
therapy degree, except for occupational therapy theory [anatomy and
physiology, special education, chemistry, Latin/classics (medical terminology), etc.]. Of course, later, when I heard about occupational therapy,
I was beyond excited! I can do ALL my passions within my profession,
and I have! I have led poetry groups in nursing homes and schools. I
have set up "Mad Scientist" camps for children with autism. I have given
lectures and seminars on the neurology of learning. I have never
designed a window display, but I have used my training to set up and
design physical environments to promote optimal learning! I needed to
find a profession that would be big enough that I wouldn't get bored
with it. Occupational therapy is said to be hard to define because it is
everything. Well, what could be cooler than that? I like having work
that needs more than a sound bite to define.

Q.   What is one thing that young people may not know about a career in occupational therapy?

A.   Occupational therapy is really a mental health profession and is the only
profession that empirically marries the brain, body, and spirit. We were
founded by a psychiatrist, a social worker, a nurse, an artist, and an architect to be able to return a person to their cherished occupations post
injury. We're very eclectic as a result of that multidisciplinary foundation,
value function beyond a healed injury, and value being engaged in one's
own valued occupation as the definition of wellness. It's a mistake to try
to put us into a box or a sound bite; we aren't a cause-and-effect discipline. If you have an occupation that you cannot engage in because of a
cognitive, emotional, or physical limitation, we can build you an on-
ramp. We blend, really, because we pay attention to and treat the fabric of
your life, the backdrop and the mundane, but if you lose those day-to-
day pieces that make your life what it is, no one can help you restore
them like an OT can. I love that. For example, I love that when I had an
injury, the lost range of motion really didn't impact my life even though
the physical therapist kept measuring that. What impacted me was I
couldn't pull my own pants up in the bathroom. I couldn't help my four-
year-old tie and untie his shoes, and I couldn't roll over in bed and kiss
my husband in the mornings or my arm would go into a spasm. The OT
not only understood that but elevated it to a priority goal and treated it
so I could return to the mundane, but important, aspects of my life.

Occupational therapists must love to solve problems and be willing to
let their hearts be opened by the sheer ecstasy of another human being
mastering a simple, but beloved, task, such as swallowing again or diaper-
ing their newborn even though a gunshot wound left them paralyzed. If

you're not willing to have your heart break open over and over by humanity, it's not the field for you. If you're looking for a protocol to follow, a cookie-cutter approach, it's not the field for you. If you want the glory of accomplishment and adoration, it's not the field for you. Our profession is designed to find deep meaning and satisfaction in the doings of others. It is a selfless profession and not for the faint of heart. People have to be creative and dedicated, or it is just too hard. They have to be able to see beyond a procedure, or it will be too abstract. They have to look beyond the deficits and see all the possibility that can be engineered for a life to be lived, fully and with joy. I love that about my profession, but some new students just see the procedures, and it's not fun for them. It's like someone focusing on the one or two sleepless nights and missing the gift of being a parent.

Q. What are the most important personal and professional qualities for people in your career?

A. Personally, people need to be resourceful and optimistic, creative, and willing to care about another person's well-being beyond fixing a concrete problem. For example, it's not enough to make sure someone can walk if they can't navigate the obstacles in the room that has their favorite sunbeam stream in the morning, where they sit with tea and the *New York Times* crossword. People have to care about that qualitative difference. It's not enough to reduce the symptoms of autism if the family still can't attend a family reunion, or be welcomed at their church on Sunday, or be part of a community and play t-ball on a team.

One's academic... Professionally, OTs need to be organized, have strong integrity, and have patience. The academic program is challenging. One has to be able to think with both sides of the brain—retain the concrete facts of science as well as apply what is learned in resourceful and creative ways. It's a real challenge for students, and a lot of them don't make it through.

Q. What are some of the pros and cons of your job?

A. Well, the big pro for me is that I can solve problems for people. I'll give you an example. Someone at my work had a client who was fixated with hair; the child couldn't move on. The staff person came to me because "you OTs can figure anything out." Of course there's no protocol for helping a child resolve a hair fixation, but we took a Curious George stuffed monkey, and a wig we had at home and stitched the hairpiece on George for the child to have and play with. We added fish gravel to make George solid and to organize the tactile sensation. How fun is that? I also was asked to look at a child who had odd stereotypical behaviors. When I observed her, I realized what she really had was a primitive reflex that wasn't integrated. We have games and playful activities for the parents that will help resolve that. I really love that trained-observer skill I have as an OT along with the science to figure out the issue and a way to make the solution fun and engaging and lighthearted.

One BIG con is that we OTs keep everything in case we will need it—all items become a potential therapeutic solution. More seriously, having to explain to others how we can contribute can become tiresome. Part of our education includes learning how to serve on interdisciplinary teams, the roles of other team members—psychologists, speech therapists, physical therapists—we spend a good bit of time teaching students how to work in those interdisciplinary teams. Other disciplines don't do this—they don't teach about occupational therapy...it's unfortunate, really; it would allow clients to get the best care. Once we do work on teams, other disciplines get a sense of what we contribute, and we can work together for a client.

One other part of being an OT that is a challenge is standing back and letting a client struggle so he or she can fully experience the victory. We call it the 'just right challenge'; to let a client struggle just enough and fail just enough that they won't lose hope but will feel the joy of success when it comes. Walking that line with a client can be hard.

I guess another con would be our tendency to blend in—what we do looks like anyone can do it, but that isn't the case— we're like that joke, why do you pay the engineer to tighten a bolt? Because she knows WHAT bolt to tighten—we're like that. Maybe others can copy what we do, but our skill is in knowing what to do, and when, to choose a specific activity to use that will engage the client, what specific aspect to address, and we have a deep tool kit to reach into to address the problem. We're team players, in general, and OTs tend to be, culturally and by training, selfless.

Q. What advice would you give to young people who are interested in becoming occupational therapists?

A. Don't go into it for the money, go into it because it will feed your soul. Do something else if you want to just earn money. Occupational therapy is too hard if you can't take pleasure in selflessly helping another do what HE wants to do, if you can't see and value the qualitative joy of another's life. And you won't ever be a great therapist; you can only be a great protocol follower. Who wants that as a best outcome? But if you love science, art, people, and problem solving, then occupational therapy just might be what you're looking for. Students in social-work programs say, "I just feel like the physical aspect of health is being overlooked," and nursing students say, "I want to be more creative and use my art," might want to look into occupational therapy. Occupational therapy students who say "this is too abstract" or who require a clear answer for each problem to be given to them so they can memorize it for the test, should look into a profession that provides that. Occupational therapy is about seeing what is needed and bringing it, not finding the pre-fab solution and fitting it to the protocol.

Q. What is the employment outlook for occupational therapists? How is the field changing?

A. One way the field is changing is that more men are entering it. I think that's a good thing. The pay is high, and that is good in many ways, but it also brings people to it that really should do something else; that worries me. The employment outlook is brisk. As long as people want to live their lives to the fullest, there will be a demand for occupational therapists.

PHARMACISTS

OVERVIEW

Pharmacists are health care professionals who provide pharmaceutical care. They take medicinal requests written by a medical provider, evaluate the appropriateness of the requests, and dispense medicine to the patient. They also spend a considerable amount of time counseling patients regarding the proper use of medicine or medical supplies, and advising them of any possible adverse side effects. A doctor of pharmacy (Pharm.D.) degree is required to practice as a pharmacist. Approximately 269,900 pharmacists are employed in the United States. Job opportunities in the field are expected to be excellent through 2018.

THE JOB

Pharmacists do more than just count pills. At retail pharmacies, they evaluate the type of medicine prescribed by your doctor, make sure the dosage is correct, check for any incompatibility with existing prescriptions, and warn people about any adverse effects. Sometimes they may contact the doctor, especially with new prescriptions, to verify the type of medicine and dosage, to suggest a generic equivalent, or to get more information from the provider. Pharmacists may compound—combine or change from a solid form to a liquid form—ingredients or medicines to create the desired prescription. This practice is rarely done today, since many medicines are now delivered in their final form by the manufacturer. However, pharmacists may add flavorings, such as fruit or bubblegum, to some juvenile medicines to make them more palatable. Most pharmacists work in community settings, such as a retail drugstore, or in a health care facility, such as a hospital or clinic.

Pharmacists are often a source of valuable health care information. They provide advice on prescription drugs and over-the-counter medications. Many people rely on their expertise regarding a variety of health care products—from the most effective eye drops to help irritated eyes to the most potent topical allergy creams. Pharmacists also provide information on other

FAST FACTS

High School Subjects
Chemistry
Mathematics

Personal Skills
Critical thinking
Judgment and decision making
Scientific

Minimum Education Level
Doctorate

Salary Range
$79,000 to $109,000 to $134,000+

Employment Outlook
Faster than the average

O*NET-SOC
29-1051.00

GOE
02.04.01

DOT
074

NOC
3131

products such as medical equipment or home health care supplies. Since they recognize the importance of total well-being, many pharmacists also provide general health advice about diet, nutrition, exercise, as well as ways to alleviate stress. Some of their duties are administrative. They maintain computerized records for customers/patients in order to avoid possible drug interactions, as well as complete insurance documents to submit for reimbursement. Pharmacists keep track of all medicine, vaccines, and other supplies, and they place orders when necessary. Some pharmacists are trained to administer vaccinations. Depending on the size of the pharmacy, they may supervise the work of pharmacy technicians, assistants, and interns. In large pharmacy departments, they manage the work of other pharmacists.

Pharmacists who are employed at hospitals or clinics often team up with other health care professionals to monitor patients' drug therapies. They may interpret medical lab results in order to design and implement the proper treatment plan, such as a nuclear medicine course or intravenous nutrition support. Often changes must be made in the type of medicine given or the dosage before obtaining the desired results. There are many pharmaceutical specialties, including the following:

Nuclear pharmacists, along with other members of a nuclear medicine team, use radioactive drugs for diagnosis and therapy of different diseases. Their duties include procuring, compounding, testing, administering, and monitoring the use of radioactive drugs such as isotopes that are used for cardiac stress tests or radioactive iodine that is used to treat certain cancers.

Nutrition support pharmacists help critically ill patients receive nutrition either by gastric tubes, by nasogastric-feeding tubes, or through intravenous feedings. They design or modify nutrition plans for patients and help them maintain optimal nutrition.

Oncology pharmacists work with *oncologists* (cancer doctors) to help design, implement, and monitor pharmacotherapeutic plans, and they make changes as needed.

Pharmacotherapists are responsible for the safe, proper, and economical use of various drugs for patient care. While they work as part of a medical professional team, they are often the primary source of drug information.

Working in consultation with other health care professionals, *psychiatric pharmacists* design and implement treatment plans for patients who have psychiatric illnesses. They make patient assessments, monitor their response to a type of drug, and identify drug-related reactions.

Managing health care information electronically and using information technology and computers is becoming an important part of pharmacy care. According to the American Society of Health-System Pharmacists, *pharmacist informaticists* "use and integrate data, information, knowledge, technology, and automation in the medication-use process for the purposes of improving health outcomes." They design and promote systems and approaches such as electronic medical records, e-prescribing, computerized prescriber order entry, bar code dispensing and administration systems, and automated dispensing cabinets.

Consulting pharmacists provide distributive, administrative, and clinical services to people in nursing facilities, prisons, psychiatric facilities, and adult day-care facilities, as well as those in their own homes. *Senior care pharmacists* are specialized consulting pharmacists who work at nursing facilities, hospices, and other long-term care facilities. They provide and oversee the implementation of drug therapy regimens for the elderly.

In addition to working at hospitals, clinics, and privately owned and chain pharmacies, pharmacists work in other settings. One example is a pharmaceutical manufacturing company. In this capacity, pharmacists conduct research to develop new drugs and test them before they are offered to the public. For example, pharmacists employed at Pfizer Inc. may be in charge of a research and development trial for a new drug to control hypertension. Working with a study group, they adjust dosages and keep track of changes in blood pressure, or any negative side effects. Once the drug passes all testing—which can take many years—pharmacists may help create and launch a marketing campaign for the new drug.

Some pharmacists choose to work for insurance companies. They are responsible for developing patient cost analysis studies, or they may help develop a new drug benefits package. Another career path is in the field of education. Pharmacists teach at colleges and universities or conduct in-service seminars and certification classes for pharmacists. Some pharmacists pursue legal training to become patent attorneys or pharmaceutical law consultants. There are also opportunities in marketing and sales.

Full-time pharmacists work about 40 hours a week, with some evening, weekend, and holiday hours required. Approximately 12 percent of pharmacists work 50 hours or more a week. Some pharmacies are open 24 hours a day; pharmacists employed at such facilities should expect to work some overnight shifts. Approximately 19 percent of pharmacists work part-time.

Pharmacists wear professional attire, often including a lab coat. Comfortable shoes are a must, since they spend the majority of their workday standing or walking to different areas of the pharmacy. Pharmacists wear gloves, masks, and other protective equipment when working with sterile products or potentially hazardous chemicals.

Attention to detail is a must for this job. Pharmacists are careful when mixing or dispensing medicine, in order to avoid costly, and potentially harmful, mistakes. Customers rely on pharmacists for advice regarding when and how to take medications, as well as potential side effects. Many times, pharmacists speak with physicians or nurses regarding a patient's prescription, either to verify a new prescription or to consult regarding generic forms of the medication. It is important for pharmacists to stay abreast of any new pharmaceutical developments as well as any changes in Medicare, Medicaid, or health insurance coverage for prescription drugs.

Some pharmacists provide consultations to different health facilities, such as nursing homes or rehabilitation centers. In such cases, a reliable means of transportation is needed in order to travel from one facility to another.

REQUIREMENTS

HIGH SCHOOL

You should take a college-preparatory track in high school that includes classes in mathematics (especially calculus and statistics) and science (especially anatomy, biology, chemistry, and physics). Additionally, you should take English and speech classes because developing good communication skills is key to success in the field. If you plan to work as a retail pharmacist or own your own drugstore, you should take business and accounting courses. Finally, taking one or more foreign languages (especially Spanish) will help you effectively interact with people who do not speak English as a first language.

POSTSECONDARY TRAINING

A doctor of pharmacy (Pharm.D.) degree is required to practice as a pharmacist. The six-year doctor of pharmacy (Pharm.D.1), the degree most commonly offered by pharmacy programs, trains pharmacists to help patients monitor chronic illnesses, to administer immunizations, and to host public education activities. There is also a postbaccalaureate degree offered—a Pharm.D.2. The American Association of Colleges of Pharmacy offers a director of pharmacy training programs at its website, www.aacp.org/RESOURCES/STUDENT/Pages/SchoolLocator.aspx.

Pharmacists who own their own businesses might augment their training in pharmaceutical science by earning a master's degree in business administration. Others earn degrees in public administration or public health.

CERTIFICATION AND LICENSING

The Board of Pharmacy Specialties, which was created by the American Pharmacists Association, offers voluntary certification in the following areas: nuclear pharmacy, nutrition support pharmacy, oncology pharmacy, pharmacotherapy, psychiatric pharmacy, and ambulatory care. The Commission for Certification in Geriatric Pharmacy also provides certification. Contact these organizations for more information about certification requirements.

All states and the District of Columbia, as well as Guam, Puerto Rico, and the U.S. Virgin Islands, require pharmacists to be licensed. Licensing requirements include earning a Pharm.D. degree from a college of pharmacy that has been approved by the Accreditation Council for Pharmacy Education and passing a series of examinations. The North American Pharmacist Licensure Exam (NAPLEX) is required by all states, U.S. territories, and the District of Columbia. The Multistate Pharmacy Jurisprudence Exam (MPJE) is required by 44 states and the District of Columbia. States and territories that do not require the MPJE have their own pharmacy law exams. The NAPLEX and MPJE are offered by the National Association of Boards of Pharmacy.

OTHER REQUIREMENTS

To be a successful pharmacist, you should have excellent communication and interpersonal skills, be very attentive to detail, have a desire to help others live healthier lives, be conscientious, have scientific aptitude, and be willing to continue to learn throughout your career.

EXPLORING

There are many ways to learn more about a career as a pharmacist. You can read books and periodicals about the field, visit the websites of college pharmacy programs to learn about typical classes and possible career paths, and ask your teacher or school counselor to arrange an information interview with a pharmacist. Professional associations also provide information about the field at their websites. For example, the Academy of Managed Care Pharmacy offers *Mapping Your Career in Managed Care Pharmacy* (www.amcp.org/mapping_your_career/contributors.cfm); the American Association of Colleges of Pharmacy offers information on pharmacy specialties (www.aacp.org), the National Association of Chain Drug Stores offers *Consider Pharmacy as a Career* (www.nacds.org/wmspage.cfm?parml=6579), and the National Community Pharmacists Association offers the *Independent Pharmacy Career Guide* (www.ncpanet.org/index.php/independent-pharmacy-career-guide). Additionally, you should try to land a part-time job at a retail pharmacy. This will give you a chance to interact with pharmacists and see if the career is a good match for your interests and abilities.

EMPLOYERS

Approximately 269,900 pharmacists are employed in the United States. Sixty-five percent work at retail pharmacies, and 22 percent are employed in hospitals. Other employers include mail-order and Internet pharmacies, pharmaceutical wholesalers, pharmaceutical manufacturers, insurance companies, offices of physicians, government agencies (including the Food & Drug Administration, Departments of Defense and Veterans Affairs, Indian Health Service, and Public Health Service), and colleges and universities.

GETTING A JOB

Many pharmacists obtain their first jobs as a result of contacts made through college internships, residency programs, or fellowships. Others seek assistance in obtaining job leads from college career services offices, newspaper want ads, and employment websites (such as RX Career Center, www.rxcareercenter.com). Additionally, professional associations, such as the American Pharmacists Association and the American Society of Health-System Pharmacists, provide job listings at their websites. See For More Information for a list of organizations. Those interested in positions with the federal government should visit the U.S. Office of Personnel Management's website, www.usajobs.opm.gov.

ADVANCEMENT

Advancement options for pharmacists vary by employment setting. Pharmacists in retail pharmacies may be promoted to the positions of pharmacy supervisor or store manager. Others become district, regional, or corporate managers. Hospital pharmacists can become supervisors or administrators. Some pharmacists go into business for themselves and open their own pharmacies. Others become professors at colleges and universities.

EARNINGS

Salaries for pharmacists vary by type of employer, geographic region, and the worker's experience level and skills. Median annual salaries for pharmacists were $109,180 in 2009, according to the U.S. Department of Labor (USDL). Salaries ranged from less than $79,270 to $134,290 or more. The USDL reports the following mean annual earnings for pharmacists by employer: health and personal care stores, $107,810; general medical and surgical hospitals, $106,210; grocery stores, $105,640; and department stores, $105,120.

Employers offer a variety of benefits, including the following: medical, dental, and life insurance; paid holidays, vacations, and sick days; personal days; 401(k) plans; profit-sharing plans; retirement and pension plans; and educational assistance programs. Self-employed workers must provide their own benefits.

EMPLOYMENT OUTLOOK

Employment for pharmacists is expected to grow faster than the average for all careers through 2018, according to the U.S. Department of Labor (USDL). Factors that are fueling demand include the growing elderly population (whose members traditionally need more prescriptions than other demographic groups), continuing scientific advances (which are creating more pharmaceutical treatment options), and the growing number of people who are becoming eligible for prescription drug coverage as a result of health care reform. The relatively small number of training programs for pharmacists is also contributing to the shortage of workers in the field.

The USDL predicts that there will be rapid employment growth at medical care establishments (such as doctors' offices, outpatient care centers, and nursing care facilities) and mail-order pharmacies. Growth will also occur at hospitals, drugstores, mass retailers, and grocery stores because pharmacists in these settings still dispense the majority of prescriptions. Pharmacists in these settings are also beginning to administer vaccinations and offer other patient care services.

The duties of pharmacists have changed in recent years. Pharmacists are spending less time dispensing drugs and more time "advising patients on drug therapies, evaluating the safety of drug therapy, administering vaccines, and counseling patients on services ranging from self-care to disease management," according to the American Pharmacists Association.

The Health Resources and Services Administration has identified some major trends in the field. It reports that more women are entering the field; they now make up half of all employed pharmacists. Women are expected to comprise 62 percent of pharmacists by 2030. Minorities are still underrepresented in the field. Only 18 percent of pharmacists were from minority groups in 2000, despite making up 25 percent of the U.S. population (as cited in the 2000 Census). Shortages of pharmacists are especially pronounced in "rural areas, low-income urban areas, and select federal institutions such as prisons."

FOR MORE INFORMATION

Visit the academy's website to read *Mapping Your Career in Managed Care Pharmacy.*
**Academy of
Managed Care Pharmacy**
100 North Pitt Street, Suite 400
Alexandria, VA 22314-3141
800-827-2627
www.amcp.org

To learn more about pharmacy education, contact
**Accreditation Council
for Pharmacy Education**
20 North Clark Street, Suite 2500
Chicago, IL 60602-5109
312-664-3575
info@acpe-accredit.org
www.acpe-accredit.org

For information on postsecondary training, contact
**American Association
of Colleges of Pharmacy**
1727 King Street
Alexandria, VA 22314-2700
703-739-2330
mail@aacp.org
www.aacp.org

For information on education, careers, and licensing, contact
American Pharmacists Association
2215 Constitution Avenue, NW
Washington, DC 20037-2907
202-628-4410
www.pharmacist.com

For information on careers and certification, contact
**American Society
of Consultant Pharmacists**
1321 Duke Street
Alexandria, VA 22314-3563
info@ascp.com
http://ascp.com

For information on careers, contact
**American Society
of Health-System Pharmacists**
7272 Wisconsin Avenue
Bethesda, MD 20814-4820
301-657-3000
www.ashp.org

For more information about pharmacy specialties, contact
Board of Pharmacy Specialties
2215 Constitution Avenue, NW
Washington, DC 20037-2907
202-429-7591
bps@aphanet.org
www.bpsweb.org

For information on state boards of pharmacy, contact
**National Association
of Boards of Pharmacy**
1600 Feehanville Drive
Mount Prospect, IL 60056-6014
847-391-4406
www.nabp.net

For information about pharmacy education and careers, contact
**National Association
of Chain Drug Stores**
413 North Lee Street
Alexandria, VA 22314-2301
703-549-3001
www.nacds.org

Visit the association's website to read the *Independent Pharmacy Career Guide.*
**National Community
Pharmacists Association**
100 Daingerfield Road
Alexandria, VA 22314-6302
800-544-7447
info@ncpanet.org
www.ncpanet.org

Interview: Linda Banares

Linda Banares, Pharm.D. is an assistant professor at Touro University College of Pharmacy in Vallejo, California, and practices as an ambulatory care clinical pharmacist at San Francisco General Hospital in San Francisco, California. She discussed her career with the editors of *Hot Health Care Careers*.

Q.   What made you want to enter this career?

A.   I have always been most drawn to the maths and sciences, and I am happiest when I am interacting with and caring for people. For these reasons, during high school I decided that I wanted to pursue a career in the health care field. I researched many professions including medicine, dentistry, dental hygiene, nursing, and pharmacy. During my senior year of high school after performing Internet searches, attending career fairs, and doing job shadowing, I came to the conclusion that pharmacy would be the best fit for me. Pharmacy appealed to me with its job security, flexibility in work hours, variety of work environments, and opportunities to care for patients while not having to do all "the dirty work" such as dealing with blood and body fluids!

Q.   What is one thing that young people may not know about a career as a health-system pharmacist?

A.   Health-system pharmacists have many more roles and responsibilities beyond counting pills and making IVs. For instance, many pharmacists spend time rounding with physicians at the patient bedside in hospitals to help select the most appropriate medications and doses based on lab values, safety, and cost. Pharmacists play key roles in facilitating medication reconciliation in hospitals, which helps to ensure that patients get on, stay on, and are discharged on their correct medications. This often involves communication with patients, their families, nurses, and providers. Many clinical pharmacists also work under collaborative practice agreements with physicians, where there is an established protocol for the pharmacist to manage medication therapy. In inpatient settings, collaborative practice will often involve high-risk medications such as anticoagulants and antibiotics. In outpatient clinic settings, the most common medications to be managed by pharmacists include those for anticoagulation, diabetes, hypertension, cholesterol, pain, and anemia.

Q.   Can you briefly describe a typical day on the job?

A.   As a clinical assistant professor at the College of Pharmacy, my time is divided between my activities as an ambulatory care pharmacist in a general medicine clinic of a large county hospital in San Francisco, and on the college campus. In clinic my primary function is to oversee/precept pharmacy students and residents on their clinical rotations. I guide them in their activities of conducting patient visits for chronic disease medication management, such as for anticoagulation, diabetes, high blood pressure, high cholesterol, and chronic pain. These activities are performed under collaborative practice agreements with the physicians, and include taking vital signs (e.g., blood pressure and heart rate), adjusting medication doses, starting or stopping medications, ordering lab tests, and educating patients on medicines and healthy lifestyle behaviors. After the patient visits, we write notes in the medical chart documenting our activities, and we submit paperwork for reimbursement of some of our services. I routinely answer drug information and insurance questions from attending physicians, medical residents, and nurse practitioners, as well as help them select the most appropriate medications for their patients based on safety, effectiveness, and cost. I also serve on several multi-disciplinary committees that focus on ongoing quality assessment and improvement of our clinic's services.

On campus I teach lectures to the pharmacy students on a variety of clinical pharmacy topics, and I help lead workshops for the students that give them hands-on experience in areas such as taking vital signs and administering immunizations. I also serve as a faculty advisor to students and serve on the curricular assessment committee of the college. In my spare time, I precept students at various community outreaches, such as health fairs where we routinely offer diabetes and high blood pressure screenings, medication education, and flu shots.

Q. What are the most important qualities for pharmacists?

A. You have to be able to get along with different personality types. No matter the pharmacy environment you end up in, you will be part of a team of people that are caring for the patient. You will need to communicate information to patients, their medical and nursing providers, and their families. You will also need to be an effective communicator with the pharmacy technicians, cashiers, and students you work with and oversee. It is crucial that you care about helping people. Multitasking comes as part of the territory with any career in the health care field, but no matter how many demands you are facing, it is always important that all activities are done with the patients' best interests in mind. In pharmacy, it is also helpful to be detail-oriented to prevent medication errors. Professionally, a strong work ethic, commitment to lifelong learning, and a willingness to give back to the profession through public policy advocacy efforts and teaching, will all serve you well.

Q. What are some of the pros and cons of your job?

A. Pros: Pharmacy offers dynamic work environments since medication treatments are always changing. There are ample opportunities to help and care for patients in a variety of work environments (inpatient, outpatient, academia, research), and in these environments there are different degrees of direct patient interaction. Good pay and job security are other benefits of pharmacy.

Cons: Pharmacists are currently not universally recognized as health care providers, which limits our ability to bill for reimbursement for cognitive (non-dispensing) services. This is something that professional pharmacy organizations are lobbying for, which would allow for justification from an economic standpoint of further expansion of clinical pharmacist roles. Another challenge is continually working to overcome common misconceptions that pharmacists' roles are limited to those of dispensing medications.

Q. What advice would you give to young people who are interested in becoming health-system pharmacists?

A. Talk to and shadow as many pharmacists in different working environ-

ments as possible. Ask their opinions on education and residency training, and where they see the future of pharmacy heading. Try to get a volunteer or paid job in a pharmacy setting so that you can see firsthand
some of the things you would be doing as a pharmacist. Get good grades
in undergraduate studies, as pharmacy school admittance is becoming
increasingly competitive. Do your research ahead of time regarding
admission requirements for colleges of pharmacy you are interested in, as
they vary from program to program. Finally, continue to pursue hobbies
to stay a well-rounded, interesting individual.

Interview: JoFlor Martinez

JoFlor Martinez is a pharmacy manager for Walgreens. She discussed her
career with the editors of *Hot Health Care Careers*.

Q.   What made you want to become a pharmacist?

A.   I became a pharmacist because it is a great career for a woman. I've
always wanted to help people and coming from a family of doctors and
nurses helped to motivate me into taking up the field as well.

**Q.   What is one thing that young people may not know about a career as
a pharmacist?**

A.   The profession of pharmacy offers employment in many different settings
such as retail (Walgreens, Osco, CVS), working in hospitals, teaching,
and research.

Q.   What are the most important qualities for pharmacists?

A.   Important personal qualities of a pharmacist are patience and having the
people skills necessary to communicate with patients, doctors, and nurses. Professionally, pharmacists should be knowledgeable about their field
and dedicated to their jobs.

Q.   What do you like most and least about your job?

A.   I enjoy meeting new people and helping everyone with their medications.
The salary is also good. My least favorite aspect is the possibility of making errors that can lead to harming the patients.

**Q.   What advice would you give to young people who are interested in
becoming a pharmacist?**

A.   I would advise young people who are interested in a career in pharmacy
to work hard and stay focused. The schooling needed to become a pharmacist is long and very competitive, but the reward is a very satisfying
career.

Q.   What is the employment outlook for your field?

A.   There are good employment prospects for pharmacists. People will
always be in need of medication to help them with various illnesses and
conditions, as well as trained professionals to dispense these medications.

PHYSICAL THERAPY ASSISTANTS AND AIDES

OVERVIEW

Physical therapy assistants and aides help physical therapists provide health care services to individuals suffering from functional problems caused by arthritis, burns, amputations, strokes, back and neck injuries, traumatic brain injuries, sprains/strains and fractures, headaches, carpal tunnel syndrome, incontinence, multiple sclerosis, cerebral palsy, spina bifida, limitations caused by old age, and work- and sports-related injuries. Physical therapy assistants are responsible for services including exercises, massages, electrical stimulation, and therapeutic baths. Physical therapy aides can assist physical therapists and assistants with simple therapy procedures but tend to have a more clerical role in the therapy team. Physical therapy assistants train for the field by earning an associate's degree

FAST FACTS

High School Subjects
Biology
Health

Personal Skills
Communication
Following instructions
Helping

Minimum Education Level
Associate's degree (assistants)
High school diploma (aides)

Salary Range
$30,000 to $48,000 to $66,000+ (assistants)
$17,000 to $23,000 to $34,000+ (aides)

Employment Outlook
Much faster than the average

O*NET-SOC
31-2021.00, 31-2022.00

GOE
10.02.02

DOT
076

NOC
6631

in physical therapy assisting; physical therapy aides learn their skills on the job. Approximately 63,800 physical therapist assistants are employed in the United States. Physical therapist aides hold about 46,100 positions. Assistants should expect very good job prospects through 2018; aides will experience strong competition for jobs.

THE JOB

People with various illnesses, diseases, or injuries often seek the help of physical therapists to help them regain strength and mobility, as well as find relief from pain. While physical therapists evaluate patients' needs and design and implement therapy programs, they turn to physical therapy assistants and aides to oversee some basic therapy procedures and much of the administrative work.

Physical therapy assistants work with patients and perform procedures as selected and supervised by physical therapists. Their patients include those with physical disabilities resulting from disease or injury or a disabling condition due to chronic illness such as arthritis, heart disease, or cerebral palsy.

When assessing a new patient, physical therapy assistants help physical therapists conduct tests and measurements to better gauge the patient's limitations. Some tests may have the patient reach or bend to determine his or her range of motion, or perhaps work with pulleys and weights to assess his or her muscle strength. Physical therapy assistants also perform gait and functional analyses to identify any weaknesses. They help patients improve their speed and adapt for many different walking surfaces and for different activities. Physical therapy assistants use gait strategies to retrain patients, especially those affected by a stroke, or teach them to use walking devices.

Physical therapy assistants help patients through a series of exercises to improve muscle strength and function. They also use therapeutic massages, both deep-tissue and surface techniques, to maintain muscle function. Physical therapy assistants administer treatments using hot or cold packs, ultraviolet and infrared lamps, or electrical stimulation equipment to improve muscle function. Traction devices and incline surfaces are also used to relieve neck or back pain. Hydrotherapy is a treatment used by physical therapy assistants to treat conditions such as osteoarthritis, osteoporosis, Parkinson's disease, or strokes. The buoyancy of the water and warmth from the pool or tub helps combat muscle stiffness and spasms or pain. Sometimes physical therapy assistants also enter the pool, especially when helping patients with water exercises.

Physical therapy assistants also help patients with cardiovascular exercises, especially those who are recuperating from a heart attack or heart surgery. Physical therapy assistants monitor patients as they go through an interval training series using recumbent bicycles, treadmills, or elliptical machines.

Physical therapy assistants also provide education and instruction. They train patients and their family members regarding the proper way to do exercises while at home. They also help patients become familiar with the use of new prosthetic or orthotic devices. Physical therapy assistants often work with other members of the patient's medical team, noting any changes or improvements in the patient's therapy progress.

Depending upon the facility and the type of physical therapy offered, physical therapy assistants may work with a variety of patients and conditions. Some physical therapy assistants work with children, those with special needs, or, in the case of a sports rehabilitation facility, they may specialize in sports-related injuries and conditions.

Physical therapy aides also help with some basic procedures, done under the direct supervision of physical therapists and assistants. They often help during hydrotherapy sessions by assisting patients into whirlpools or tubs, or even entering the pool as patients do their exercises. Aides also apply hot and cold packs to soothe tightened muscles and use paraffin baths to relieve patients' pain from arthritis, bursitis, or other chronic joint inflammation. Some aides are trained to give massages and other such treatments. They prepare patients for their treatments, including helping them undress (if necessary), removing supportive devices such as braces and slings, and getting them properly situated on machinery.

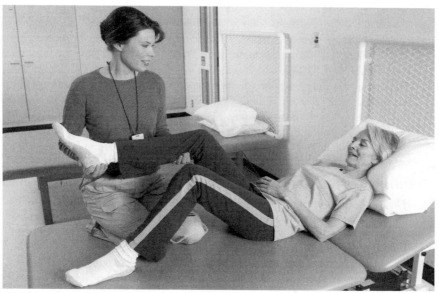

Employment for physical therapy assistants and aides is expected to grow by 35 percent from 2008 to 2018, according to the U.S. Department of Labor. (Hemera Technologies/ Thinkstock)

A large part of their job is composed of clerical duties. Aides often maintain the front office, including answering the phone, greeting and processing patients as they enter the facility, and filling out insurance forms or other paperwork. They keep track of supplies and equipment and reorder these materials when necessary.

Aides also clean and maintain treatment areas, including hydrotherapy pools and spas, and request necessary repairs. They often transport patients from one area of the facility or hospital to another, sometimes moving patients in wheelchairs or other equipment.

Full-time assistants and aides typically work 40 hours a week. Shifts vary depending on the facility and its patient load—some evening and weekend hours should be expected in order to accommodate patients' schedules and needs.

Many physical therapy assistants and aides wear scrubs, smocks, or other clothing that allows easy movement. Assistants and aides wear bathing suits when helping patients engaged in water therapy exercises. Comfortable, skid-resistant shoes are a must, since a great part of their day is spent standing or walking with patients.

REQUIREMENTS

HIGH SCHOOL

In high school, take anatomy and physiology, biology, health, physics, chemistry, social sciences, computer science, physical education, English, and speech classes.

POSTSECONDARY TRAINING

Physical therapy assistants train for the field by earning an associate's degree in physical therapy assisting, which is required by most states as one of the criteria for licensing. The Commission on Accreditation in Physical Therapy Education (www.apta.org/CAPTE), which accredits postsecondary physical therapy assistant programs, has accredited more than 260 educational programs. Students complete both classroom and clinical instruction. Typical classes include Introduction to Physical Therapy, Medical Terminology, First Aid and CPR, Applied Kinesiology, Human Anatomy and Physiology, Principles of Biological Science, and Patient Management. Physical therapy aides do not need a college degree. They learn their skills through on-the-job experience and training.

CERTIFICATION AND LICENSING

Most states require physical therapy assistants to hold a license, certification, or registration to work. Requirements for most states include graduating from an accredited educational program and passing the National Physical Therapy Exam. Visit the Federation of State Boards of Physical Therapy website, www.fsbpt.org, for more information about licensure/certification requirements. Physical therapy aides do not need to be certified or licensed.

OTHER REQUIREMENTS

Physical therapy assistants and aides need to be in good physical condition to work with patients of all ages and sizes as they undergo procedures and exercises. Oftentimes, they must kneel, stoop, walk, or otherwise physically assist patients during sessions.

It is important for physical therapy assistants and aides to have good interpersonal skills, especially when working with patients who may be suffering from injury or pain. They should be patient and have compassion for their patients. Other important traits include the ability to follow instructions, good organizational skills, a detail-oriented personality, and an interest in helping others.

EXPLORING

There are many ways to learn more about a career as a physical therapist assistant or aide. You can read books (such as *Introduction to Physical Therapy for Physical Therapist Assistants,* by Olga Dreeben-Irimia) and journals about the field (such as *Physical Therapy,* which is published by the American Physical Therapy Association, APTA), visit the websites of college physical therapy assisting programs to learn about typical classes and possible career paths, and ask your teacher or school counselor to arrange an information interview with a physical therapist assistant or aide. Professional associations can also provide information about the field. The APTA, the leading physical therapy association in the United States, provides a wealth of information on education and careers at its website, www.apta.org. You should also try to land a part-time job in a setting where physical therapists, assistants, and aides are employed. This will give you a chance to interact with physical therapy professionals and see if the career is a good fit for your interests and abilities.

EMPLOYERS

Approximately 63,800 physical therapist assistants are employed in the United States. Physical therapist aides hold about 46,100 positions. They work in hospitals, clinics, offices of physicians and other health care professionals, inpatient and outpatient rehabilitation facilities, skilled nursing homes, fitness centers, sports facilities, corporate or industrial health centers, pediatric centers, elementary and secondary schools, colleges and universities, and private homes.

GETTING A JOB

Many assistants and aides obtain their first jobs as a result of contacts made through career fairs, college internships, or networking events. Others seek assistance in obtaining job leads from college career services offices, newspaper want ads, and employment websites. Additionally, the American Physical Therapy Association provides job listings and career planning resources at its website, www.apta.org/applications/careercenter.aspx. Those interested in positions with the federal government should visit the U.S. Office of Personnel Management's website, www.usajobs.opm.gov.

ADVANCEMENT

With further college education, physical therapist assistants can become physical therapists. Aides can become assistants and eventually physical therapists. Other means of advancement include salary increases, taking on managerial duties, or becoming a college professor at a physical therapy education program.

EARNINGS

Median annual salaries for physical therapist assistants were $48,290 in 2009, according to the U.S. Department of Labor. Salaries ranged from less than $30,400 to $66,460 or more. The median annual salary for physical therapy aides was $23,890. Ten percent earned less than $17,330, and 10 percent earned more than $34,100.

Employers offer a variety of benefits, including the following: medical, dental, and life insurance; paid holidays, vacations, and sick and personal days; 401(k) plans; profit-sharing plans; retirement and pension plans; and educational-assistance programs. Part-time workers must provide their own benefits. Approximately 28 percent of physical therapy assistants and aides work part-time.

EMPLOYMENT OUTLOOK

Employment for physical therapist assistants and aides is expected to grow much faster than the average for all careers through 2018, according to the U.S. Department of Labor (USDL). The growing population (especially elderly people who need rehabilitation services); breakthroughs in medical technology and treatments that are allowing more babies to survive serious birth defects and people to survive illnesses and injuries; and the aging of the large Baby Boomer population, which will require an increasing amount of cardiac and physical rehabilitation, will create very good employment prospects. Aides will face a more competitive labor environment due to an abundance of workers in the field. The USDL reports that employment opportunities should be particularly strong in acute hospital, skilled nursing, and orthopedic settings—areas that treat a large number of elderly patients.

FOR MORE INFORMATION

For detailed information on education and careers, contact
American Physical Therapy Association
1111 North Fairfax Street
Alexandria, VA 22314-1488
800-999-2782
www.apta.org

For information on accredited programs, contact
Commission on Accreditation in Physical Therapy Education
accreditation@apta.org
www.apta.org/CAPTE

Interview: Mary Knerr

Mary Knerr is a physical therapist assistant. She has been employed by Advocate Good Samaritan Hospital in Downers Grove, Illinois, for 21 years. Mary discussed her career with the editors of *Hot Health Care Careers*.

Q.   What made you want to enter this career?

A.   There were a number of reasons that made me want to enter this career, but I believe I can trace back my initial interest to the therapy sessions that I accompanied my brother to after his serious car accident. He sustained a number of fractures, including vertebral fractures that required extensive back therapy. I volunteered at a local hospital to further investigate the profession and thought the job seemed very diverse—everything from athletes in sports rehab to geriatric patients who needed help after a stroke. The thought of helping people in a real way was very appealing.

Q.   What is one thing that young people may not know about a career as a physical therapist assistant (PTA)?

A.   One thing that young people may not know about a career as a PTA is the true scope of the practice. PTAs may choose to do wound care, treating non-healing wounds or burns. They may choose to work with newborns in a neonatal intensive care unit or children born with physical handicaps in a clinical or school setting. They could work in an acute-care setting, where you treat patients who have recently had heart surgery, joint replacement, or multiple traumatic injuries. There is acute rehab, where you can train spinal cord injury patients to be as independent as possible or help a stroke patient regain use of affected muscles. If the geriatric population is their preference, then subacute rehabilitation in skilled nursing facilities may be desirable.

Q. What are the most important qualities for PTAs?

A. The personal and professional qualities that are most important for this career include: (1) Patience: you may be dealing with patients who are critically ill or in a great deal of pain, and you must be patient and flexible when treating them or interacting with their family members. (2) Problem solving: you must draw upon your experience and knowledge and sometimes the specialized knowledge of coworkers to plan how best to help a patient. (3) Good communication skills: therapists regularly interact with patients and their families, doctors, nurses, social workers, speech therapists, and occupational therapists. Communication is vital to keep abreast of a patient's medical status and to know how effective treatment has been. (4) Friendliness/ability to put people at ease: Illness and injury can be very frightening to people, and they will always respond better to therapists who are friendly and confident.

Q. What do you like most and least about your job?

A. What I like most about my job are my coworkers. I am fortunate enough to work with a group of highly skilled, dedicated therapists who have camaraderie and a sense of humor that I truly appreciate.

What I like least about my job is encountering people that I am unable to help because of the extent of their medical problems. Many times their family and friends do not have reasonable expectations and believe that recovery is always possible. These patients and their families may try to pressure the therapist to continue treatment beyond what is feasible, and this can cause serious dilemmas.

Q. What advice would you give to young people who are interested in the field?

A. The advice that I would give someone who is interested in this career would be to volunteer in a hospital or clinic to see if the job is right for you or to apply for a job as a physical therapy aide to get more exposure to patients and therapists.

Q. What is the employment outlook for PTAs?

A. The employment outlook for this field is very bright indeed. Several calls/week and five to 10 mailings/week looking to hire PTAs are quite common. I have had many students of mine find a job in a desirable setting within days of graduation.

PHYSICAL THERAPISTS

OVERVIEW

Physical therapists, also known as *physiotherapists,* provide health care services to individuals suffering from functional problems caused by arthritis, burns, amputations, stroke, back and neck injuries, traumatic brain injuries, sprains/strains and fractures, headaches, carpal tunnel syndrome, incontinence, multiple sclerosis, cerebral palsy, spina bifida, limitations caused by old age, and work- and sports-related injuries. They evaluate, design, and implement individualized programs to help reduce pain, improve mobility, and increase the quality of life for patients of all ages. Physical therapists use many different techniques for their work including exercise equipment, massage, and electrotherapy. A minimum of a post-baccalaureate degree in physical therapy is required to work in the field. Approximately 185,500 physical therapists are employed in the United States. Employment for physical therapists is expected to grow much faster than the average for all careers through 2018.

THE JOB

Many individuals suffer from functional limitations due to injury, disease, surgery, advanced age, or other medical conditions. Their limitations may include difficulty in walking, problems shifting weight, a limited range of motion in their arms or legs, a weak grip, or even decreased endurance. Physical therapists provide therapy services to help patients eliminate or reduce these problems. They also develop and implement therapy programs to help people retain their mobility and flexibility and generally have a healthy lifestyle.

When working with a new patient, physical therapists must first evaluate the individual. They conduct a physical assessment to gauge the patient's physical condition and limitations, as well as a short interview to learn more about the patient's lifestyle, work habits, degree of pain, degree of mobility, and therapy goals. Oftentimes, physical therapists consult with other health care professionals such as doctors, nurses, speech-language pathologists, audiologists, dentists, and social workers, as well as members of the patient's family, to complete the assessment. Once a diagnosis of the patient's movement dysfunction is made, physical therapists design a therapy plan to suit the patient's capabilities and schedule. Therapy plans, depending on the extent of the patient's disability or injury, can include a series of exercises, muscle manipulation and massage, traction, hot or cold therapy, ultrasound, and electrotherapy. Physical therapists use many different tools and techniques to achieve positive results such as hand weights, exercise balls and bands, risers, and cardiovascular equipment (treadmills, stationary bicycles, etc.).

Many physical therapists specialize in a specific clinical area and may implement therapy plans that are customized to meet different needs and goals. Patients suffering from cardiopulmonary disease or those who have undergone recent cardiac or pulmonary surgery often have decreased endurance or lung function. For example, physical therapists use manual therapy to help remove excess secretions from the lungs, or they use chest mobilization exercises to increase lung capacity.

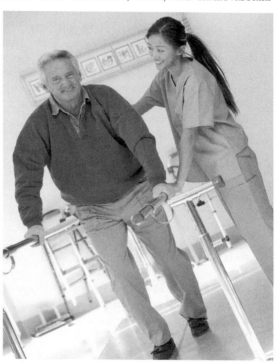

A physical therapist helps a patient re-learn how to walk. The U.S. Department of Labor predicts that more than 56,000 new jobs will be available for physical therapists through 2018. (BananaStock/Thinkstock)

Physical therapists often work with elderly patients who have arthritis, osteoporosis, balance disorders, joint replacements, or Alzheimer's disease. Techniques used with geriatric patients include water aerobics, stretching exercises, and light weight lifting to improve their mobility. Physical therapists also teach geriatric patients better ways to conduct daily activities, such as the proper way to safely climb and descend stairs or how to use a walker or other aid.

Pediatric physical therapy is another specialty. When working with infants, children, and young adolescents, physical therapists create a plan to address not only areas of concern, but also the capabilities and attention spans of their young patients. Infants needing physical therapy may be those born with a congenital disorder such as spina bifida. Physical therapists may suggest leg braces or specific exercises and massages to keep limbs flexible and avoid contracting. Children with developmental delays also benefit from physical therapy. For example, balls and other squeezable toys may be incorporated into an exercise plan to increase mobility and strength.

Orthopedic physical therapy, the most common and identifiable specialty, treats patients suffering from injuries sustained at home, on the athletic field, or at the workplace as well as those needing rehabilitation after orthopedic surgery. Most orthopedic therapy is conducted on an outpatient basis. For a patient recovering from a sports injury to a muscle in his or her arm, for example, physical therapists may use techniques such as therapeutic exercises, hot or cold packs, and even electrotherapy to expedite neuromuscular stimulation and retraining. They may use arm pulleys or resist-a-bands to increase strength. Continuous passive motion machines can be used to increase a patient's rotator cuff flexibility and strength.

Physical therapists are responsible for charting their patients' scheduled therapy sessions and progress. They consult with other health care professionals to keep them abreast of the patient's progress or to discuss or update them regarding changes in therapy plans. Depending on their employer, physical therapists may also complete and submit billing sheets for services rendered, maintain equipment, and order supplies and equipment.

The work of physical therapists is physically demanding. They spend a considerable amount of time each day standing, stooping, walking, bending, reaching, lifting, and operating equipment or using various tools.

A normal workweek for a full-time physical therapist is 40 hours, with time off on weekends or holidays. However, many physical therapists have some weekend and evening hours in order to accommodate patient loads. Approximately 27 percent of physical therapists work part-time. Some travel may be necessary, especially for those providing home health therapy.

Physical therapists may be required to wear a uniform, which often consists of hospital scrubs, pants, and smock, and comfortable, non-skid shoes.

REQUIREMENTS

HIGH SCHOOL

In high school, take science courses (especially anatomy, biology, chemistry, and physics), as well as classes in mathematics, statistics, physical education, social science, psychology, computer science, English, and speech. If you plan to work in an area with a large number of people who do not speak English as a first language, you should take a foreign language—especially Spanish.

POSTSECONDARY TRAINING

A minimum of a post-baccalaureate degree in physical therapy from an accredited physical therapy program is required to work in the field. The Commission on Accreditation of Physical Therapy Education (www.apta.org/CAPTE), which accredits entry-level academic programs in physical therapy, has accredited 212 education programs. Nine of these programs award master's degrees, and 203 award doctoral degrees. Typical courses in a doctorate program include Introduction to Physical Therapy, Gross Human Anatomy, Physiology, Functional Histology, Neuroanatomy, Joint Function and Movement, Biophysics, Clinical Applications, Psychosocial Theory and Practice, Musculoskeletal Dysfunction, Neuromuscular Dysfunction, Cardiopulmonary Dysfunction, Applied Pathophysiology, Case Management in Physical Therapy Practice, and Clinical Fieldwork.

Aspiring physical therapy students can use the PT Centralized Application Service (www.ptcas.org), which allows one to apply to multiple accredited physical therapy programs at one time.

CERTIFICATION AND LICENSING

Certification, while voluntary, is highly recommended. It is an excellent way to stand out from other job applicants and demonstrate your abilities to prospective employers. The American Board of Physical Therapy Specialities offers certification in the following specialties: cardiovascular and pulmonary, clinical electrophysiology, geriatrics, neurology, orthopaedics, pediatrics, sports physical therapy, and women's health. Contact the board for more information.

All states require physical therapists to be licensed. Licensing requirements vary by state but typically include graduation from an accredited physical therapy education program; passing the National Physical Therapy Examination, which is administered by the Federation of State Boards of Physical Therapy (www.fsbpt.org); and fulfilling state requirements (which may involve passing additional examinations).

OTHER REQUIREMENTS

Physical therapists must be in optimum physical condition in order to lift patients and assist them in turning, standing, or walking. A positive disposition is also helpful when working with patients who may be suffering from chronic pain or limited mobility. Physical therapists must often motivate their patients during therapy sessions, and this is best done with a smile and encouraging words. Other important traits include compassion, an interest in helping others, and good time-management skills.

EXPLORING

There are many ways to learn more about a career as a physical therapist. You can read books and journals about the field (such as *Physical Therapy*, which is published by the American Physical Therapy Association, APTA), visit the websites of college physical therapy programs to learn about typical classes and possible career paths, and ask your teacher or school counselor to arrange an information interview with a physical therapist. Professional associations can also provide information about the field. The APTA, the leading physical therapy association in the United States, provides a wealth of information on education and careers at its website, www.apta.org. You should also try to land a part-time job in a setting where physical therapists are employed. This will give you a chance to interact with physical therapists and see if the career is a good fit for your interests and abilities.

EMPLOYERS

Approximately 185,500 physical therapists are employed in the United States. About 60 percent of physical therapists work in hospitals or in offices of health practitioners. Employment opportunities also exist at nursing homes, home health services providers, outpatient care centers, adult day-care programs, industrial settings, schools, and government agencies (such as the Department of Defense and Veterans Affairs and the Indian Health Service). Other physical therapists work as professors and researchers at colleges and universities. Some have their own businesses. In fact, the American Physical Therapy Association reports that nearly 22 percent of physical therapists are owners of, or partners in, a physical therapy practice.

Books to Read

Krumhansl, Bernice. *Opportunities in Physical Therapy Careers.* New York: McGraw-Hill, 2005.

Lais, Toni. *Career Diary of a Physical Therapist.* New York: Garth Gardner Company, 2008.

Pagliarulo, Michael A. *Introduction to Physical Therapy.* St. Louis: Mosby, 2006.

GETTING A JOB

Many physical therapists obtain their first jobs as a result of contacts made through college internships, clinical experiences, or networking events. Others seek assistance in obtaining job leads from college career services offices, newspaper want ads, and employment websites. Additionally, the American Physical Therapy Association provides job listings at its website, www.apta.org/applications/careercenter.aspx. Those interested in positions with the federal government should visit the U.S. Office of Personnel Management's website, www.usajobs.opm.gov.

ADVANCEMENT

At large therapy providers, physical therapists may advance to managerial and supervisory positions. Others may start their own businesses and offer their services on a contract basis to hospitals, nursing facilities, and other therapy providers.

EARNINGS

Salaries for physical therapists vary by type of employer, geographic region, and the worker's experience level and skills. Median annual salaries for physical therapists were $74,480 in 2009, according to the U.S. Department of Labor (USDL). Salaries ranged from less than $52,170 to $105,900 or more. The USDL reports the following mean annual earnings for physical therapists by employer: home health care services, $83,500; nursing care facilities, $78,990; offices of physicians, $77,120; offices of other health practitioners, $75,760; and general medical and surgical hospitals, $75,030.

Physical therapists usually receive benefits such as health and life insurance, vacation days, sick leave, and a savings and pension plan. Self-employed workers must provide their own benefits.

EMPLOYMENT OUTLOOK

Employment for physical therapists is expected to grow by 30 percent through 2018, according to the U.S. Department of Labor—or much faster than the average for all careers. Factors that are fueling growth include an increasing elderly population, which has a strong need for physical therapy services; changes in insurance reimbursement, which will allow more people to have access to physical therapy services; the implementation of the Individuals with Disabilities Education Act, which ensures that disabled students will have better access to physical therapy and other rehabilitative services in schools; and advances in medicine and technology that are allowing people with severe trauma, serious illness, and birth defects to survive, which will create the need for more physical therapists to treat these patients.

Physical therapists who specialize in treating the elderly will have especially strong job prospects. Typical employers for these workers include acute care hospitals, skilled nursing facilities, and orthopedic settings. Opportunities will also be good in rural areas, where there is a shortage of trained physical therapists.

FOR MORE INFORMATION

For information on education and careers, contact
American Physical Therapy Association
1111 North Fairfax Street
Alexandria, VA 22314-1488
800-999-2782
www.apta.org

For information on accredited programs, contact
Commission on Accreditation in Physical Therapy Education
accreditation@apta.org
www.apta.org/CAPTE

Interview: Steven W. Forbush

Steven W. Forbush, PT, Ph.D. is an assistant professor of physical therapy at the University of Central Arkansas in Conway, Arkansas. He discussed his career and the field of physical therapy with the editors of *Hot Health Care Careers*.

Q. What made you want to enter this career?

A.   I was in a pre-medical program in my undergraduate school, majoring in biology and minoring in chemistry and psychology. I was planning on going into some form of medical-based field and was thinking of dentistry. I then realized I didn't want to spend my life with my hands in other person's mouths. I had already decided I didn't want to be a doctor as I did not want to prescribe medicine, or have life and death decisions weighing on me at critical times. Some of my classmates (ones I respected) had decided on going on with physical therapy programs, and I decided to look into this field in the summer between my junior and senior years. I met a gentleman in my hometown who was in private practice (men were not common in the profession at that time and private practice was also an unusual setting) in physical therapy and was doing well. I already had all of the prerequisite courses to apply and decided this was where I wanted to be. After 25 years in the profession, I went back to school to gain a Ph.D. in physical therapy so I could continue to advance the profession through the educational realms.

Q.   What do you like most and least about your career?

A.   I am really excited about my field and my career, even after over 30 years of working in this area. I enjoy knowing that I am making an immediate, and sometimes a life-long, difference in my patient's lives. I also am now able to improve the skills and knowledge of students at my DPT program and established therapists through other continuing education offerings so that they may influence the lives of countless other patients and clients. I am truly excited to go to work each and every day and daily learn more to become a better therapist and person through my patient and peer interactions. I also enjoy being active in the American Physical Therapy Association and its components as this is the only organization representing the profession of physical therapy and its interests on a state or federal level.

I don't enjoy watching all the medical professions protect turf in every legislative session rather than working together to improve all aspects of health care. I also don't enjoy fighting for continuing payment for the services we provide as a profession through the constant cost-cutting that is occurring on the state and federal levels.

Q.   What is the one thing that young people may not know about a career in physical therapy?

A.   I am not sure the public really understands the field of physical therapy and all that it offers. I have people come up to me all the time and, after I tell them I am a physical therapist, suggest they need a massage, have other misconceptions they relate to me, or suggest that they would like to see me but feel they need to see a physician first to find out what is wrong with them. Young persons (and old persons in the general public) do not understand that our profession should be the profession to visit for any neurological, musculoskeletal, or other functional or movement problem they may have. Very few of the problems anyone experiences in their lifetime are from a serious pathology...and if these pathologies are present, the physical therapist is trained to recognize that the problem needs to be addressed by another medical specialty and refer them accordingly.

Q.   Can you please tell us about your program?

A.   The University of Central Arkansas, where I am now a professor, offers a Doctor of Physical Therapy Program, which is the program that is the expected program for a graduating physical therapist anywhere in the United States. It is a full three-year program encompassing 126 graduate credit hours of education, including 43 hours of clinical practicum, in order to graduate. To get into a typical physical therapy program (including our's) one needs to have 48 credit hours of specific undergraduate pre-requisite courses to prepare them for the program. Most programs around the U.S. are very similar to ours, and all programs must be accredited through the same national body, the Commission on Accreditation in Physical Therapy Education.

Q.   What type of students pursue study—and find success—in your program?

A.   The typical person finding their way to physical therapy as a profession is relatively academically gifted (average entrance GPA in our program is a 3.73, with a science GPA of 3.53), usually like the field of biology, have an altruistic interest and wish to help others, are relatively social and can interact and communicate well with persons of all ages, and usually have had some connection to the field of physical therapy in their life history. If a person is willing to accept change and adapt to a constantly changing environment and is service oriented in the typical business model, they will be even more successful. I like the student who is willing to smile, politely challenge what is told to them, be willing to admit they are wrong, and be humble in the process.

Q.   What advice would you offer physical therapy majors as they graduate and look for jobs?

A.   I am very active in advising new graduates on jobs and areas of interest as they graduate. Almost every student has an area where they have found the most reward as they have worked through their varied practicum experiences, and I always suggest they start and stay in the area where they have the most passion. I suggest they find a workplace with ethical and work standards that most closely resembles their own; a setting where they will have the proper mentorship to continue to grow; a setting in the area of the country where they are eager to live and work; and a setting where they will be challenged on a regular basis. Jobs are available in almost any setting, in almost any town with a population over 25,000, and in almost any region in the country so job scarcity is rarely an issue.

Q.   What is the employment outlook for physical therapy? Have certain areas of this field been especially promising (or on the decline) in recent years?

A.   Physical therapy is consistently rated as one of the fastest-growing professions with one of the highest demands in the medical arena. In the past 30 years there has only been one short period of time when supply of physical therapists has exceeded the demand of the society (just after the passage of the BBA in 1997, which greatly limited the payments for any rehabilitative professionals) and this self-corrected within less than five years. The population of the U.S. has been aging according to all statistics and this demographic typically needs more rehabilitative care than other areas of the population. The population is also participating in more youth-based organized competitive sport (leading to more acute and chronic injury), getting heavier (leading to more joint and muscle problems), and living a more sedentary lifestyle in middle age (also a predictor for more pain complaints), and all of these predict a greater need for a group of professionals specializing in neuromusculoskeletal differential diagnosis and persons specialized in the correction of movement disorders. Also, the state and federal governments have emphasized care of children in all the medical payment systems leading to a rapid growth in the field of pediatric physical therapy.

Interview: Jennifer Zaleskie

Jennifer Zaleskie, PT, DPT is a physical therapist at Burke Rehabilitation Hospital in White Plains, New York. She discussed her career with the editors of *Hot Health Care Careers*.

Q.   Can you tell us a little about Burke Rehabilitation Hospital?

A.   Burke is a 150-bed hospital that specializes in treating physical disabilities, including stroke, brain injuries, spinal cord injuries, Parkinson's disease and other neurological disorders, cardiac disease, chronic pulmonary disease, arthritis, orthopedics, joint disease, and amputation. The Burke team is dedicated to helping individuals regain a maximum level of mobility and independence following a disabling illness or injury.

Q.   How long have you worked in the field?

A.   I am a new professional, working as a physical therapist for almost two years. However, I have been very active within the profession and professional association for more than six years since beginning graduate school. My involvement with the American Physical Therapy Association (APTA) and Student Assembly offered me many wonderful opportunities and great networking resources.

Q.   What made you want to enter this career?

A.   When I was 14 years old, I sustained an injury doing gymnastics that required surgery. This began my first exposure to physical therapy. After a couple months of therapy, which helped me regain my strength and flexibility, I was able to return to competitive gymnastics. At this point, I knew I was interested in pursuing physical therapy as a future career. Like many starting out, I wanted to be an orthopedic sports physical therapist to potentially work with athletes and athletic teams. As my knowledge of physical therapy expanded throughout school, I learned about all the other specialties within the field of physical therapy. This led me to my love for rehabilitation, more specifically neurological rehabilitation (i.e. spinal cord injury, brain injury, stroke).

Q.   What is one thing that young people may not know about a career in physical therapy?

A.   When "physical therapy" is mentioned, typically many people automatically think of orthopedics or sports injuries. There is so much more to the profession than sports/orthopedic-based physical therapy. Physical therapists work in various settings such as pediatric clinics, schools, hospitals, operating rooms, rehabilitation hospitals, with sports teams, geriatrics, etc. Although hands-on clinical care is the majority of what physical therapists do, there are also non-clinical positions to include administration roles, teaching, and political/lobbyist positions.

Q. What are the most important qualities for physical therapists?

A. Successful physical therapists possess the seven core values of professionalism as defined by the American Physical Therapy Association: accountability, altruism, compassion/caring, excellence, integrity, professional duty, and social responsibility. These attributes are constantly being developed throughout one's educational and professional career.

Q. What advice would you give to aspiring physical therapists?

A. The best way to learn more about physical therapy is to volunteer or intern at a local clinic, hospital, rehabilitation center, etc. There is also a lot of useful information on the student section of the APTA website for high school and undergraduate students, which can be found at www.apta.org/students.

Q. What are the best ways to find a job?

A. Right now, physical therapists are in demand. Many new grads apply for a position at one of their clinical affiliation sites. On average, a physical therapy student will be required to complete four to six clinical affiliations in various practice settings throughout their education. In addition to reinforcing what is learned in the classroom, expanding clinical skills, and improving critical thinking, the clinical affiliations give student physical therapists an opportunity to determine what type of setting he or she would like to practice in upon graduation.

The American Physical Therapy Association also has a "Job Bank" on its website, which is an excellent way to search for/find a job. It is a search engine that lists opportunities available in various settings, locations, positions desired, and so on. Visit www.apta.org/applications/careercenter.aspx for more information.

PHYSICIAN ASSISTANTS

OVERVIEW

Physician assistants (PAs) provide medical care that ranges from basic primary health care to specialty and surgical procedures. They work under the supervision of physicians. Physician assistants work in almost all medical and surgical specialties and in every medical setting. Nearly 25 percent of PAs specialize in family/general medicine, according to the American Academy of Physician Assistants (AAPA). Other popular practice areas include surgical subspecialties (22.4 percent) and internal medicine subspecialties (10.8 percent). Associate, baccalaureate, and master's degree programs in physician assisting are available; 80 percent of accredited programs offer the option of a master's degree. According to the AAPA, there are more than 74,450 practicing physician assistants in the United States. Employment for physician assistants is expected to grow much faster than the average for all careers through 2018.

THE JOB

The emergency room is filled to capacity, with many more patients waiting to be triaged. A boy with a possible broken arm, an elderly woman with a bad case of the flu, and a young woman having an asthma attack are just a few of the cases that the emergency room staff is facing. With the help of a physician assistant, patients with less-critical cases are seen, diagnosed, treated, and, hopefully, sent home. Physician assistants play an important role in these situations. They help speed the flow of patients through the emergency department. But PAs don't just work in emergency rooms. Wherever there are patients in need of health services, there are physician assistants to provide key support to physicians.

PAs are trained to provide diagnostic, therapeutic, and preventive health care services, working under the supervision of physicians. When taking a new case, they take into account the patient's medical history—what medicines the patient is currently taking, his or her family medical history, and all presenting symptoms and complaints. They give the patient a complete examination and, depending on the patient's symptoms, order blood work or other laboratory tests such as x-rays, MRIs, or CT scans. With such information, PAs are able to make a diagnosis and begin to treat the patient's condition. PAs prescribe the proper medication or refer the patient to a physician for further evaluation. PAs can prescribe medications in all 50 states, the District of Columbia, Guam, and the Commonwealth of the Northern Mariana Islands. In the majority of employment settings, prescriptions and laboratory test requests written by the PA must be evaluated and approved by the attending medical physician. PAs working in the inner city or in a rural setting may not be constantly supervised by a physician. They sometimes may be the sole care provider in the clinic. Such settings may have physicians present only some days of the week or for only a few hours a day. In these cases, the PA is responsible for seeing patients and conferring with medical physicians as needed or as dictated by state law.

PAs also practice preventive health care services by counseling patients about health care issues. They may caution patients on potential side affects or adverse reactions from certain medications. When diagnosing a patient with hypertension, for example, a PA may give nutritional advice such as limiting salt intake, changing dietary habits, and participating in cardiovascular exercise, as well as continuing to take prescribed medications.

PAs can also perform certain procedures, depending on their area of specialty. When working in an orthopedic practice setting, for example, PAs can apply a splint to a badly sprained finger or cast a fractured elbow. In a pediatric setting, PAs can suture a child's facial laceration. PAs working in a dermatological office can perform procedures ranging from wart excisions to medical and cosmetic Botox injections, as well as lipodissolve treatments.

Many PAs choose to practice in a surgical setting. When conducting pre-operative care, PAs take patient histories, record vital signs, and handle other tasks that prepare the patient for the surgical procedure. During major surgery, PAs may work as the first or second assistant to the surgeon. Their duties, depending on the type of surgery, could include completing a vein harvest or placing indwelling catheters and tubes such as Foley catheters, intravenous lines, or arterial lines. They may also be called upon to assist in the closure of the surgical incision. PAs may also be responsible for post-operative care of their patient. Duties include the insertion or removal of lines and catheters and chest tubes or changing dressings and bandages. PAs also answer questions from patients and their families regarding the patient's status after the surgery.

Nursing homes, assisted-living communities, and long-term rehabilitation centers are other settings in which PAs practice. In these settings, PAs conduct weekly or monthly assessments of geriatric patients (many of whom have chronic conditions); monitor prescription medicines, nutrition, or any needed inpatient therapy; and order outpatient services or tests. They start treatment on any new illnesses or injuries common with their patients' age group, such as pneumonia, pressure sores, heart problems, or even dementia. If working with patients in rehab, PAs monitor the types of exercise programs used or track the progress of therapy sessions. Some PAs, especially those working in rural areas, may make house calls. Whether making a monthly patient assessment at a nursing home, a house visit, or daily rounds at a hospital, PAs must report back to their attending physician and give their findings and recommendations.

PAs also have administrative duties. Charting—writing or electronically recording information regarding the patient's conditions, findings, and any recommended treatment—is part of the job, no matter the physician assistant's specialty. Some PAs are responsible for ordering the office or clinic's medical supplies or equipment such as stethoscopes, syringes, vaccines, drugs, and culture kits. They meet with drug representatives or medical supply salespeople to discuss new drugs and equipment. Some PAs, especially those working in a large clinical practice, train and supervise medical technicians and assistants.

Full-time physician assistants work about 40 hours a week, including evenings, weekends, and overnight shifts.

REQUIREMENTS

HIGH SCHOOL

Recommended high school classes include those in anatomy and physiology, biology, chemistry, mathematics, English, speech, computer science, health, psychology, nutrition, the social sciences, and statistics.

POSTSECONDARY TRAINING

There are nearly 160 physician assistant training programs in the United States that are accredited by the Accreditation Review Commission on Education for the Physician Assistant (www.arc-pa.org). Associate, baccalaureate, and master's degree programs in physician assisting are available. The American Academy of Physician Assistants reports that the average PA program takes 26.5 months to complete. Typical courses in the first year of study include Anatomy and Physiology, Biochemistry, Clinical Laboratory, Clinical Medicine, Medical Ethics, Microbiology, Pathology, and Pharmacology. Second-year classes include Emergency Medicine, Family Medicine, Geriatric Medicine, Internal Medicine, Obstetrics/Gynecology, Orthopedics, Pediatrics, Psychiatry, Radiology, and Surgery. Students also complete clinical rotations in these various practice areas. The Physician Assistant Education Association offers a list of programs at its website, www.paeaonline.org. It also offers the Central Application Service for Physician Assistants, a Web-based application service that allows students to apply to more than one program by using the same application. Visit https://portal.caspaonline.org for more information.

Physician assistants can also attend postgraduate educational programs in internal medicine, surgery, pediatrics, neonatology, rural primary care, emergency medicine, and occupational medicine.

CERTIFICATION AND LICENSING

All states and jurisdictions require physician assistants to pass the Physician Assistant National Certifying Examination, which is administered by the National Commission on Certification of Physician Assistants. Applicants must have graduated from an accredited physician assistant training program. Those who become certified can use the title, physician assistant-certified.

Did You Know?

From 2008 to 2018, nine of the top 20 jobs that are adding the most positions that require an associate's degree or postsecondary vocational award are in the health care industry. They are:

✔ Registered Nurses: +582,000 jobs

✔ Nursing Aides: +276,000 jobs

✔ Licensed Practical Nurses: +156,000 jobs

✔ Dental Hygienists: +63,000 jobs

✔ Radiologic Technicians and Technologists: +37,000 jobs

✔ Medical Records and Health Information Technicians: +35,000 jobs

✔ Medical and Clinical Laboratory Technicians: +25,000 jobs

✔ Massage Therapists: +23,000 jobs

✔ Surgical Technologists: +23,000 jobs

Source: U.S. Department of Labor

OTHER REQUIREMENTS

Hospital and clinical settings often include many different health care workers. PAs must be team players and be able to work with a variety of workers and personalities. They should have excellent communication skills to interact well with patients and coworkers. Since medical technology is ever changing, PAs must be willing to continue to learn throughout their careers. They often attend seminars, conventions, or continuing-education classes as a requirement for licensure. Other important traits for physician assistants include emotional stability, the ability to make decisions under pressure, a desire to serve others, and compassion for people who are in pain or other discomfort.

EXPLORING

There are many ways to learn more about a career as a physician assistant. You can read books and magazines about the field, visit the websites of college physician assisting programs to learn about typical classes and possible career paths, and ask your teacher or school counselor to arrange an information interview with a physician assistant. Professional associations can also provide information about the field. The American Academy of Physician Assistants provides information on education and careers at its website, www.aapa.org/about-pas. You should also try to land a part-time job in a medical office. This will give you a chance to interact with physician assistants and see if the career is a good fit for your interests and abilities.

EMPLOYERS

There are more than 74,450 practicing physician assistants in the United States, according to the American Academy of Physician Assistants (AAPA). The AAPA reports that more than 37 percent of physician assistants work at hospitals. Other major employers include single-specialty groups, 24.2 percent; multi-specialty physician groups, 11.2 percent; solo physician practices, 8.6 percent; and community health centers, 4.7 percent.

GETTING A JOB

Many physician assistants obtain their first jobs as a result of contacts made through college internships or clinical rotations, career fairs, or networking events. Others seek assistance in obtaining job leads from newspaper want ads, college career services offices, and employment websites. Additionally, the American Academy of Physician Assistants provides job listings at its website, www.aapa.org/find-a-job. Those interested in positions with the federal government should visit the U.S. Office of Personnel Management's website, www.usajobs.opm.gov.

ADVANCEMENT

Physician assistants advance by receiving pay raises and managerial responsibilities. Some pursue postgraduate education and become specialists in internal medicine, emergency medicine, and other areas. Other physician assistants continue their education to become physicians or college professors.

EARNINGS

Salaries for physician assistants vary by type of employer, geographic region, and the worker's experience, education, and skill level. Salaries for physician assistants ranged from less than $55,880 to $115,080 or more in 2009, according to the U.S. Department of Labor.

Full-time clinically practicing PAs had mean annual incomes of $93,105 in 2009, according to the American Academy of Physician Assistants. In 2008, PAs earned the following mean annual salaries by practice area: emergency medicine, $87,251; surgical subspecialties, $78,879; dermatology, $78,418; pediatric subspecialties, $76,136; and general surgery, $75,988.

Physician assistants usually receive benefits such as health and life insurance, vacation days, sick leave, and a savings and pension plan. Part-time workers must provide their own benefits.

EMPLOYMENT OUTLOOK

Employment for physician assistants is expected to grow much faster than the average for all careers through 2018, according to the U.S. Department of Labor (USDL). Physician assistants are in strong demand as a result of the growing U.S. population and the health care industry's attempts to contain costs (physician assistants are a cost-effective alternative to physicians). Opportunities will be best in rural and inner-city health care facilities. In addition to jobs in traditional office-based settings, the USDL reports that an increasing number of opportunities will be available in hospitals, public clinics, academic medical centers, and prisons.

FOR MORE INFORMATION

For more information on educational programs and careers, contact
American Academy of
Physician Assistants
950 North Washington Street
Alexandria, VA 22314-1552
703-836-2272
aapa@aapa.org
www.aapa.org

For information on certification, contact
National Commission on
Certification of Physician
Assistants
12000 Findley Road, Suite 200
Duluth, GA 30097-1409
678-417-8100
nccpa@nccpa.net
www.nccpa.net

For information on accredited educational programs, contact
Physician Assistant
Education Association
300 North Washington Street,
Suite 710
Alexandria, VA 22314-2544
703-548-5538
info@paeaonline.org
www.paeaonline.org

Interview: Kara D. Larson

The editors of *Hot Health Care Careers* discussed the career of physician assistant with Kara D. Larson, MSPAS, PA-C a physician assistant and the vice president (2009-2010) of the Student Academy of the American Academy of Physician Assistants.

Q. What made you want to enter this career?

A. I wanted to practice medicine since my seventh-grade life science course. That was the easy decision; the hard decision was what medical career was right for me. Going into college, I labored over the decision between a nursing or pre-med major. After much time comparing both fields, I realized I was more interested in the medical decision-making of taking care of a patient and chose pre-med.

When I graduated from college, I again was faced with a tough decision: medical school or physician assistant (PA) school. Both programs are fundamentally the same, learning multiple disease processes and their treatment while assimilating the vast number of patient skills. I chose to become a PA instead of a M.D., not because I couldn't handle the rigors of medical school, but because of the difference in lifestyle I would have as a PA.

Becoming a PA takes 2.5 years after college whereas becoming an M.D. takes four years after college for medical school and then three to seven years of residency before you are prepared to enter the medical field. This shorter time frame for PA school, with a corresponding lower amount of student loans for repayment, made the profession very attractive to me. I had the ability to start working with a practice as well as start my family sooner without being overwhelmed with large loan repayments.

Another attractive aspect of the PA profession is the flexibility to work in various medical specialties. An M.D. must decide in medical school what specialty he will devote his entire life to, whereas a PA has the ability to work in different specialties throughout his career. Also, the PA shares the pressure of being the "final decision-maker." A PA works within the medical team, making decisions together with the M.D. and always has the ability to consult with his supervising physician for final decisions.

Q. What is one thing that young people may not know about a career as a physician assistant?

A.   Young people may have encountered PAs in the primary care fields (family practice, pediatrics, women's health) as their health care providers. Therefore, they may not be aware that PAs practice in such diverse specialties as emergency medicine, internal medicine, neurology, dermatology, multiple surgical specialties, and many others. Numerous fields are open to PAs, leading to a wonderful career in which you will never be bored!

Q. If you could do anything differently in preparing for your career in college/high school, what would it be?

A.   I would shadow PAs in various specialties for a better understanding of the flexibility of PAs throughout the medical field. I didn't understand this flexibility (a great plus for the profession) until I was on clinical rotations during PA school.

Q. Can you please briefly describe a day in your life on the job?

A.   I work in a family medicine/urgent care office with two physicians and two other PAs. We work 12-hour shifts, with two days on and two days off. I begin my day by looking over lab and x-ray reports from my last shift, determining if a patient needs to return to discuss lab results and have more testing or if the nurse on duty should notify the patient of normal results.

At 8 A.M. patients are triaged and placed in exam rooms. Our office does not take appointments, so I never know the next problem I will encounter, and I spend the next 12 hours treating complaints ranging from sore throat to chest pain to prescription refills, charting as I go. I see all ages of patients—ranging from the youngest to the oldest. I spend the day determining when labs and x-rays should be ordered and interpreting those results as well as writing numerous prescriptions for antibiotics, diabetes and high blood pressure medicine, and pain medicine.

As a part of the practice we see many urgent-care cases, so I get lots of opportunities to suture lacerations, cast broken bones, and drain abscesses. I work alongside my supervising physician but have autonomy in my work. The M.D. is there for help when I need it for a difficult patient scenario, but I am not required to have his approval for my plan or to have him sign my chart or prescriptions. I may go through the entire day without needing consultation or may have several complicated patients requiring his assistance. In these cases, we always work as a team, making the best decision together. Though I have a large amount of autonomy during the day, I must always remember one of the most important pieces of information I learned in PA school: "Know what you don't know and when you need help." At the end of a normal day I've seen and treated 20-30 patients. I'm tired, but I always finish with the overwhelming satisfaction of having made a difference.

Q.   What are the most important personal and professional qualities for people in your career?

A.   Compassion is the number-one quality for all PAs. Compassion is the source of all other qualities exhibited by the best PAs. It is the guide during the difficult days of school when you feel like giving up the overwhelming task of learning the mountain of medical information. It is the quality that spurs you into studying and reading so you can provide the best information to your patients, and it is the quality that endears your patients to you.

Q.   What are some of the pros and cons of your job?

A.   Pros:

✔   Having the amazing responsibility to guide patients and help them make life-changing decisions (a pro because of the amazing privilege).

✔   Building a relationship with a patient and his/her family.

✔   Working in a growing profession—it's only headed up!

✔   The availability to work in multiple specialties. M.D.s must decide in medical school which specialty they will work in for the rest of their lives; however, PAs are free to navigate the medical field and work in any specialty (family practice, neurology, surgery, etc.), with only on-the-job training required.

Cons:

✔   Having the amazing responsibility to guide patients and help them make life-changing decisions (a con because of the stress involved in decision making).

Did You Know?

Physician assistants in Mississippi earned the highest mean annual income ($112,093) in 2008, according to the American Academy of Physician Assistants. Other top-paying states for physician assistants include Delaware ($105,083), Alaska ($105,071), Nevada ($103,609), California ($102,144), and Connecticut ($100,958). The three lowest-paying states were North Dakota ($81,358), Pennsylvania ($82,001), and South Dakota ($82,421).

✔ Long hours and very busy days. There is a shortage of medical providers, which leads to pressure to see a large number of patients per day, leading to less comprehensive care.

✔ Jobs in certain specialties are limited by the number of physicians who are entering the field, since PAs must work in a team with physicians.

Q. What advice would you give to young people who are interested in becoming physician assistants?

A. Study hard, and work harder! Due to the small number of PA schools compared to medical schools, as well as the exponential growth of the profession, admission is very competitive.

Shadow multiple PAs in various specialties and settings (i.e., hospital and outpatient) to understand how PAs function. The PA role is variable based on specialty. The family-practice PA is relatively autonomous, whereas the surgical PA may work closer to his supervising PA in the surgical setting.

If possible, work as a medical assistant or patient care technician in a hospital. This is not the most glamorous job (it involves bed changes and patient baths), but it will give you a glimpse into the health care setting as well as teach you basic skills. You will be ahead of your classmates if you already know how to take vital signs (blood pressure, pulse, respirations), start IVs, and perform blood-draws. This experience will help you develop one of the most important skills in medicine—patient assessment. Patient assessment is the ability to determine the overall condition of a patient with simple observation of external signs (i.e., the subtlety of determining breathing difficulty and ill-appearing features of patients). This skill cannot be taught; it is developed with experience.

PHYSICIANS

OVERVIEW

Physicians, also known as *doctors,* assess, diagnose, and treat patients of all ages and with many different conditions. Their methods of treatment may include prescribing medications and diagnostic tests, offering counseling on nutrition and exercise, and conducting surgery and other medical procedures. Many physicians specialize by focusing on a particular system, a part of the body, or particular age group. A medical degree is necessary to enter the field. Approximately 661,400 physicians are employed in the United States. Employment opportunities for physicians should be very good through 2018.

THE JOB

Physicians play an important role in our society. We rely on their knowledge of medical technology and treatment methods to help us when we are sick, or in order to stay healthy. There are two types of physicians: the designation, M.D., for Doctor of Medicine, and D.O., for Doctor of Osteopathic Medicine. M.D.s, also known as *allopathic physicians,* use surgery and drugs to treat patients, while D.O.s, also known as *osteopaths,* practice holistic patient care in addition to prescribing medicine and surgery. They pay special attention to the body's musculoskeletal system when examining patients and stress preventive medicine.

Physicians diagnosis illnesses, prescribe medications, and/or administer treatments. Sometimes they perform diagnostic tests to help confirm a diagnosis or refer patients to a *medical specialist* (such as an *oncologist* if they suspect that a

FAST FACTS

High School Subjects
Biology
Health

Personal Skills
Communication
Critical thinking
Helping
Judgment and decision making
Scientific

Minimum Education Level
Medical degree

Salary Range
$51,000 to $173,000 to $700,000+

Employment Outlook
Faster than the average

O*NET-SOC
29-1061.00, 29-1062.00,
29-1063.00, 29-1064.00,
29-1065.00, 29-1066.00,
29-1067.00, 29-1069.01,
29-1069.02, 29-1069.03,
29-1069.04, 29-1069.05,
29-1069.06, 29-1069.07,
29-1069.08, 29-1069.09,
29-1069.10, 29-1069.11,
29-1069.12, 29-1069.99

GOE
14.02.01

DOT
070

NOC
3112

A Statistical Snapshot of 2009
Medical School Applicants and Enrollees

✔ 42,269 people applied to medical school—a slight increase over the 42,231 applicants in 2008.

✔ Fifty-two percent of applicants and enrollees were male.

✔ Seven percent of enrollees were African American—the largest percentage since 1999.

✔ The number of Latino applicants declined by 1 percent, and the number of enrollees in this group also declined (but only very slightly).

✔ The number of Native American applicants declined by 5 percent from 2008 to 2009, and the number of enrollees decreased by 11 percent during that same time period.

Source: American Association of Medical Colleges

patient has cancer) or laboratory for additional testing. Physicians may see patients suffering from injuries or pain, and they perform procedures ranging from suturing lacerations, to setting broken bones, to prescribing medications to help alleviate pain and discomfort. Physicians also counsel patients on health and may suggest dietary or lifestyle changes to improve their patients' conditions.

Some physicians are *primary care doctors,* providing a wide range of general services. They often have a group of long-term patients that they see on a regular basis. Primary care doctors see patients for a variety of reasons including wellness care, routine physicals and immunizations, and the treatment of minor injuries, infections, or diseases. If the patient has more specific health needs, primary care physicians will then refer him or her to a specialist. Some examples of primary care doctors are those practicing *family and general medicine, internal medicine,* and *pediatrics. Family and general medicine practitioners* are typically the first physician practitioners an individual sees when ill or injured. They diagnose and treat a wide variety of illnesses or injuries—from broken bones, to the flu, to respiratory infections. *General internists* treat problems that affect the internal organ systems, such as the liver, stomach, kidneys, and digestive tract. *General pediatricians* provide health care services to infants, children, teens, and young adults.

Physician specialists are trained to focus on a particular system or part of the body. Some specialties, especially those involving surgery or other procedures, require additional training during residency or fellowship. Specialists work with primary care doctors in treating patients for a particular medical condition, or for complete care throughout life. Examples of medical specialties include *neurology, obstetrics and gynecology, anesthesiology,* and *orthopedic surgery.*

The following paragraphs detail some of the largest medical specialties:

Anesthesiologists are specially trained in anesthesia and peri-operative medicine. They treat patients before, during, and after surgery or any other medical procedure that requires anesthesia. Before a surgery begins, anesthesiologists assess the patient and consult with the surgical team to create an anesthesiology plan customized for the patient's needs. They take into account airway management and provisions for pain management. During surgery, they administer anesthesia and monitor the patient's vital life functions—heart rate, blood pressure, body temperature, and breathing. After surgery, they make sure the patient is stabilized and monitor him or her for any adverse reactions to the anesthesia.

Dermatologists treat conditions and diseases of the skin, scalp, hair, and nails. They treat patients suffering from conditions ranging from acne to cancerous lesions.

Emergency medicine physicians, also known as *emergency room physicians,* are specially trained to care for patients with illnesses or injuries that require immediate medical attention. Emergency medicine covers the field of general medicine, but it also involves practically all fields of medicine, surgery, and surgical sub-specialties. Emergency medicine physicians diagnose, treat, and stabilize patients with conditions ranging from lacerations to heart attacks. They may also treat patients suffering from injuries caused by sports or trauma (such as a car accident or a gunshot wound). Some emergency physicians also train staff members regarding cardiopulmonary resuscitation, advanced cardiac life support, and advanced trauma life support. Some participate in mock disaster drills with other health care professionals in order to be ready when a real emergency occurs.

In the 1990s, a movement to introduce medical professionals who focused solely on the care of hospital inpatients began. These physicians are known as *hospitalists.* Since that time, there has been much debate about whether their existence is a good thing. But one thing is certain: their numbers are growing, from approximately 800 in 1990 to 30,000 today, partly due to the increasing number of people admitted to hospitals nationwide and partly due to the movement to reform health care. Hospitalists are doctors who work only in hospitals. They take over for primary care physicians or internists who have to juggle their inpatient and outpatient workloads. In addition to patient care, hospitalists handle administrative tasks such as ordering tests and medications and ensuring that their orders are carried out correctly, filling out paperwork that details patient care, and overseeing patient discharge. Approximately "82.3 percent of practicing hospitalists are trained in general internal medicine, 6.5 percent in general pediatrics, 4 percent in an internal medicine subspecialty, 3.7 percent in family practice, 3.1 percent in internal medicine pediatrics, and 0.4 percent in a pediatrics subspecialty," according to the Society of Hospital Medicine.

Obstetricians and gynecologists (OB/GYNs) are responsible for the general health of women. They also provide care related to pregnancy and the reproductive system. OB/GYNs give patients annual physicals and important tests such as Pap smears or breast exams. They try to catch early occurrences of cancer in the breast, cervix, or reproductive system. OB/GYNs also specialize in prenatal care, delivery, and postnatal care.

Most Women Surgeons Love Their Careers

More than 82 percent of women surgeons surveyed by Dr. Kathrin M. Troppmann of the University of California-Davis Medical Center and her colleagues said that they would choose surgery as a career path again if given the chance. Slightly more than 77 percent of male surgeons said they would choose the profession again.

Despite these findings, a career as a surgeon involves significant lifestyle challenges. The survey found that "the profession is associated with high degrees of patient acuity, significant on-call responsibility, and irregular work hours, all requiring a significant commitment of personal time." The survey's authors point out that many accommodations have been put in place to encourage women to pursue careers in this male-dominated field. Here are a few other interesting findings from the survey:

✔ More than 83 percent of female surgeons would recommend surgery as a career path to young women.

✔ The most popular specialty among both sexes was general surgery (39.3 percent of women and 46.7 percent of men practiced in this area).

✔ Women surgeons worked a median of 60 hours per week; men worked 65 hours.

✔ A higher percentage of women surgeons than men felt that there should be more part-time work options for surgeons.

✔ More female than male surgeons believed that maternity leave was important and that child care should be available in the workplace.

Dr. Troppmann and her colleagues surveyed 895 surgeons who were board certified in 1988, 1992, 1996, 2000, or 2004. Women made up 20.3 percent of respondents.

Psychiatrists are trained in the study and treatment of mental disorders. Their patient assessment includes a mental status examination and compilation of case history. Diagnostic tests may be prescribed, including neuroimaging and other neurophysiological techniques. Psychiatrists can prescribe treatments such as medication, psychotherapy, or transcranial magnetic stimulation. Depending on the severity of the patient's condition, treatment can be conducted during hospitalization or on an outpatient basis.

Radiologists are specially trained to take and interpret medical images. Through the use of x-rays, radioactive substances, sound waves, or the body's natural magnetism, radiologists can determine the presence and severity of injuries and diseases. Some radiologists sub-specialize in a particular area of the body or system, such as head and neck radiology or breast imaging. Others sub-specialize in interventional radiology, which allows them to treat patients with minimally invasive interventional techniques. Angioplasty, angiography, stent placement, and biopsy procedures are some examples of interventional radiology techniques.

Surgeons specialize in the treatment of injury or disease through surgical procedures. Physicians perform general surgery or may specialize in surgery on a specific area of the body or system. For example, *orthopedic surgeons* perform procedures related to the musculoskeletal system, *neurosurgeons* specialize in surgical procedures on the brain and nervous system, and *cardiothoracic surgeons* specialize in conducting surgeries on the chest, heart, and lungs. Other surgical specialists include *otolaryngologists* (treatment and surgery for conditions or injuries to the ear, nose, and throat) and *plastic or reconstructive surgeons*.

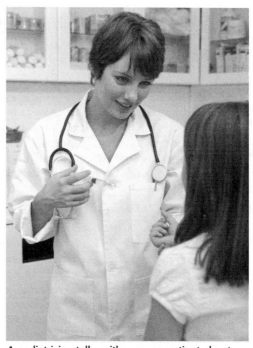

A pediatrician talks with a young patient about proper nutrition. (Jupiterimages/Thinkstock)

Physicians, regardless of their specialty, have additional duties including charting patients' progress and treatments; consulting with other physicians, health care workers, and patients and their families; and participating in staff meetings. Depending on the size and scope of their medical practice, some physicians may be responsible for other office management duties including billing, staff education, and administrative tasks. Some physicians, especially those employed by university or teaching hospitals, may supervise, train, and mentor medical students, interns, and residents. Some physicians also teach at medical schools or conduct scientific research and publish their findings in medical journals or other scholarly publications. Physicians sometimes provide expert testimony in legal proceedings.

Physicians work in hospitals, private offices, or clinics. Certain specialties, such as family medicine, pediatrics, or obstetrics/gynecology, lend themselves to private practice, while others—such as radiology, emergency medicine, and urology—are practiced in physician groups, hospitals, or other health care settings.

Physicians work in clean and sterile conditions. Their uniform consists of either hospital scrubs and gown, or other professional attire. They are often aided by a staff of other health care professionals such as nurses, physician assistants, nurse aides, therapists, technicians, and medical secretaries. Their days are often stressful; physicians can expect to work with multiple patients with varying degrees of illness.

Many physicians work long and irregular hours. More than 40 percent of all doctors working in the United States log 50 or more hours a week, including evening, weekend, and holiday hours. Depending on their specialty, physicians are "on call" day and night and deal with many patient complaints or emergencies outside the office.

REQUIREMENTS

HIGH SCHOOL

You will need to study for many years before you can become a physician. In high school, take a college-preparatory track that includes as many science classes as possible (especially chemistry, biology, and anatomy and physiology), as well as courses in mathematics, computer science, psychology, English, speech, foreign languages (especially Latin), and social studies.

POSTSECONDARY TRAINING

A medical degree is necessary to enter the field. Preparation for this career is very demanding. Medical students must complete eight years of training after high school, plus three to eight years of internship and residency. Applying to and succeeding in medical school can be challenging. Aspiring medical students must also take and pass the very demanding Medical College Admission Test (www.aamc.org/students/applying/mcat), a national examination that is administered by the Association of American Medical Colleges (AAMC). To assist students in this process, the AAMC has developed a useful publication, *The Road to Becoming a Doctor,* which can be accessed by visiting www.aamc.org/students/considering.

Approximately 65 percent of medical school applicants major in biology or another physical science at the undergraduate or graduate levels. Others major in pre-med.

More medical schools are reaching out to students with nonscience backgrounds, including those in the humanities, according to *Newsweek.* For example, 40 percent of students recently accepted to the University of Pennsylvania's medical school had nonscience backgrounds. By accepting students from nonscience backgrounds, medical schools are trying to create more well-rounded students "who can be molded into caring and analytical doctors."

There are 129 medical schools accredited by the Liaison Committee on Medical Education, which accredits M.D. medical education programs. The American Osteopathic Association (AOA) accredits colleges that award a D.O. degree. The AOA has accredited 25 schools in 31 locations.

According to the AAMC, a typical medical school curriculum is as follows: Year 1—biochemistry, cell biology, medical genetics, gross anatomy, structure and function of the organ systems, neuroscience, and immunology; Year 2—infectious diseases, pharmacology, pathology, clinical diagnoses and therapeutics, and health law; Years 3 and 4—generalist core (family and community medicine, obstetrics and gynecology, surgery, etc.), neurology, psychiatry, subspecialty segment (anesthesia, dermatology, orthopedics, urology, radiology,

Cancer Doctors in Short Supply

The growing elderly population (who are often more susceptible to certain types of cancer), a rising number of cancer survivors, and a large number of predicted retirements by oncologists is expected to create a shortage of these medical specialists by 2020, according to a study by the American Society for Clinical Oncology's Workforce Implementation Working Group. In fact, the Group predicts a shortage of up to 4,080 oncologists by 2020. In addition to encouraging more physicians to pursue careers in oncology, the Group suggests the following steps to alleviate the predicted shortage: encouraging existing oncologists to continue to practice past the typical retirement age, improving the efficiency of oncologists via technology, and increasing the use of other health care professionals (such as general practitioners, physician assistants, and nurse practitioners) in oncology-related settings.

ophthalmology, otolaryngology), continuity-of-care segment (sub internships, emergency room and intensive-care experiences), and electives.

As they approach their fourth year of school, medical students choose a specialty area in which they want to practice and begin applying to graduate medical education programs, which are known as residencies. Students obtain residencies through the National Resident Matching Program. Residencies can last anywhere from three to seven years depending on the specialty.

Students who plan to conduct biomedical research often attend joint M.D./Ph.D. programs. In these programs, which typically last seven or eight years, students learn the research skills that will help them as scientists and the clinical skills that will allow them to practice medicine. Visit www.aamc.org/students/considering/exploring_medical/research/mdphd to learn more about M.D./Ph.D. dual degree training.

Medical school tuition is high. The AAMC reports that "annual tuition and fees at state medical schools in 2008-2009 averaged $23,581 for state residents and $43,587 for non-residents. At private schools, tuition and fees averaged $41,225 for residents and $42,519 for non-resident students." Housing and living expenses were not included in these figures. A number of private and government financial aid programs are available to help students pay for medical school. Visit the websites of the associations in the For More Information section for details.

CERTIFICATION AND LICENSING

Physicians can earn voluntary board certification in a variety of medical specialties. They must participate in medical residencies and pass an examination by a member board of the American Osteopathic Association or the American Board of Medical Specialties.

Once they complete their medical training, physicians must take an examination in order to be licensed to practice medicine. Licensing is required in all 50 states and U.S. territories. The board of medical examiners in each state administers the examinations.

OTHER REQUIREMENTS

Physicians must be able to think quickly and clearly and must stay calm—especially when dealing with patient emergencies. Good bedside manners are a must—meaning physicians should have empathy toward their patients' conditions, be good listeners, and be able to have a kind and sincere disposition when counseling patients and their families.

EXPLORING

There are many ways to learn more about a career as a physician. You can read books about the field. Here is one suggestion: *White Coat Wisdom,* by Stephen J. Busalacchi (Apollo's Voice, 2008). You can also visit the websites of medical schools to learn about typical classes and medical specialties, and you can ask your teacher or school counselor to arrange an information interview with a physician or talk to your doctor about his or her career. Professional associations also provide information about the field. The American Medical Association provides a wealth of information at its website, www.ama-assn.org. The Association of American Medical Colleges (AAMC) also offers two useful websites: Considering a Medical Career (www.aamc.org/students/considering) and AspiringDocs.org (www.aspiringdocs.org), which aims to increase diversity in medicine. The AAMC also offers an annual career fair for students who are interested in learning more about careers in medicine. Visit the AAMC website for more information. You should also try to land a part-time job in a doctor's office. This will give you a chance to interact with physicians and see if the career is a good fit for your interests and abilities.

EMPLOYERS

Approximately 661,400 physicians are employed in the United States. About 53 percent of physicians and surgeons work in medical offices. Nineteen percent are employed by hospitals. Other physicians are employed by government agencies, schools, correctional facilities, and outpatient care centers. Approximately 12 percent are self-employed.

According to the American Medical Association, the following medical areas employed the most physicians: internal medicine, 20.1 percent; family medicine/general practice, 12.4 percent; pediatrics, 9.6 percent; obstetrics and gynecology, 5.6 percent; anesthesiology, 5.5 percent; psychiatry, 5.2 percent; general surgery, 5.0 percent; and emergency medicine, 4.1 percent.

GETTING A JOB

Many physicians obtain their first jobs as a result of contacts made during their residencies. Others seek assistance in obtaining job leads from medical school career services offices, newspaper want ads, and employment websites. Some professional associations, such as the American Academy of Family Physicians, provide job listings at their websites. See For More Information for a list of organizations. Job listings can also be found at the *Journal of the*

American Medical Association's website, www.jamacareercenter.com. Some new graduates start their own solo private practices, enter into a partnership with other physicians, or enter into a group practice. Those interested in positions with the federal government should visit the U.S. Office of Personnel Management's website, www.usajobs.opm.gov.

ADVANCEMENT

Physicians advance by assuming managerial duties, becoming well-known for their medical skills, by becoming experts in their medical specialty, or by opening their own practices. Some physicians become medical administrators or college professors.

EARNINGS

Salaries for physicians vary by type of employer, geographic region, and the employee's experience level, specialty, and skills. The U.S. Department of Labor (USDL) reports the following mean annual earnings for physicians by specialty in 2009: anesthesiology, $271,264; family and general practice, $167,245; internal medicine, $181,081; obstetrics/gynecology, $279,635; pediatrics, $126,955; psychiatry, $149,866; and general surgery, $219,770. Mean annual salaries for physicians and surgeons, not otherwise classified were $173,860 in 2009. Some physicians earned less than $51,750. Top specialists can earn much higher salaries. For example, very experienced plastic surgeons can earn more than $700,000.

While work in these careers is lucrative, earnings are offset by high medical malpractice insurance and the higher-than-average number of hours worked. For example, OB/GYNs worked an average of 2,637 hours a year, according to the USDL—much higher than the average of 2,008 annual hours for all workers.

Employers offer a variety of benefits, including the following: medical, dental, and life insurance; paid holidays, vacations, and sick and personal days; 401(k) plans; profit-sharing plans; retirement and pension plans; and educational assistance programs. Physicians who own their own practices or who are in a partnership with other doctors must provide their own benefits.

EMPLOYMENT OUTLOOK

Employment opportunities for physicians should be very good through 2018. In fact, the U.S. Department of Labor predicts that 144,100 new jobs will become available for physicians from 2008 to 2018.

The rapidly growing U.S. population, the predicted doubling of the number of people over age 65 between 2000 and 2030, rising expectations about the quality and ready availability of health care services, an aging physician workforce, the increasing availability of health insurance as a result of health insurance reform, and a trend toward reduced hours for physicians has created a potential physician shortage in coming years, according to the Association of American Medical Colleges (AAMC).

To address this shortage, the AAMC recommends that enrollment at U.S. medical schools be increased by 30 percent (or 5,000 students annually) by 2015. The Association says that this goal can be accomplished by increasing enrollment at existing schools and by founding new allopathic medical schools.

Physicians who are willing to work in rural and low-income areas will have the best job prospects. Opportunities will also be good for physicians who specialize in caring for the elderly because this segment of the population is growing rapidly and its members require more medical care than people in other demographics.

FOR MORE INFORMATION

For information on accredited post-M.D. medical training programs in the United States, visit the council's website.
Accreditation Council for Graduate Medical Education
515 North State Street, Suite 2000
Chicago, IL 60654-4865
www.acgme.org

For information on family medicine, contact
American Academy of Family Physicians
PO Box 11210
Shawnee Mission, KS 66207-1210
fp@aafp.org
www.aafp.org

To read the *Osteopathic Medical College Information Book,* and for information on careers and financial aid, visit the AACOM website.
American Association of Colleges of Osteopathic Medicine (AACOM)
5550 Friendship Boulevard, Suite 310
Chevy Chase, MD 20815-7231
301-968-4100
www.aacom.org

For information on board certification, contact
American Board of Medical Specialties
222 North LaSalle Street, Suite 1500
Chicago, IL 60601-1117
www.abms.org

For comprehensive information on medical education and careers, contact
American Medical Association
515 North State Street
Chicago, IL 60654-4854
800-621-8335
www.ama-assn.org

For information on osteopathic medicine, contact
American Osteopathic Association
142 East Ontario Street
Chicago, IL 60611-2864
800-621-1773
www.osteopathic.org

For information on accredited medical schools in the U.S. and Canada, contact
Association of American Medical Colleges
2450 N Street, NW
Washington, DC 20037-1126
202-828-0400
www.aamc.org

Bureau of Health Professions
U.S. Department of Health and Human Services
5600 Fishers Lane, Room 8A-09
Rockville, MD 20857-0002
http://bhpr.hrsa.gov

For information about the career of hospitalist, contact
Society of Hospital Medicine
1500 Spring Garden, Suite 501
Philadelphia, PA 19130-4070
800-843-3360
www.hospitalmedicine.org

Interview: Victor DeJesus

Dr. Victor DeJesus is a board-certified physician in internal medicine who currently works in private practice. He discussed his career with the editors of *Hot Health Care Careers*.

Q. What made you want to enter this career?

A. My father's death due to an abdominal wound affected me greatly and was my motivation in becoming a doctor. At a young age, I envisioned myself someday becoming a doctor with the skills and knowledge to prevent such an untimely death and spare other families the bitter pain of losing a loved one.

Q. What is one thing that young people may not know about a career as a physician?

A. It's not a walk in the park. A doctor's job can never be nine to five. Our responsibility to each patient continues even after the office visit. We get called any time of the day and as a solo practitioner, even an out-of-town vacation doesn't spare me from patient demands and frantic calls from my office staff.

Q. What are the most important qualities for physicians?

A. I believe that perseverance and a good memory are the two most important qualities that a medical student should possess to finish medical school. Once in private practice, a doctor who shows sincere compassion and attentiveness to the patients' needs will surely be rewarded with a good patient following and a financially stable practice.

Q. What do you like most about your job?

A. The actual patient care experience is my biggest fulfillment. Seeing my patients' quality of life improve is the best feeling I can ever get.

Q. What advice would you give to young people who are interested in becoming physicians?

A. The practice of medicine is a lifetime commitment with more challenges than ever: (1) lower insurance reimbursements with more cuts in the near future; (2) unpredictable work schedules and long working hours; (3) malpractice lawsuits, which can potentially wipe out all life savings; (4) a steep learning curve for the business part of the practice; and (5) a gloomy outlook on the horizon with the federal government's new health care reform. However, an aspiring doctor who can accept these challenges as part of the job and sees fulfillment in making people's lives better should pursue this career.

Q. What is the employment outlook for physicians?

A. Medical doctors need not worry about job security. With President Obama's plan of adding another 30 million Americans to the ranks of the insured, there is a plenty of work for every doctor in every field of medicine. In fact, the American Medical Association confirms a large physician shortage in the field of primary care (pediatrics, family medicine, and internal medicine) and projects the use of more physician extenders, such as nurse practitioners and physician assistants, to improve patient flow and prevent a crisis.

RADIOLOGIC TECHNICIANS AND TECHNOLOGISTS

OVERVIEW

Radiologic technicians operate and maintain x-ray machinery and equipment, while *radiologic technologists* perform more complicated diagnostic imaging procedures such as magnetic resonance imaging scans and computed tomography scans. They are sometimes referred to as *radiographers*. Educational requirements vary by specialty, but radiologic technicians and technologists typically require education ranging from a certificate to a bachelor's degree to enter the field. Approximately 286,800 radiologic technicians and technologists are employed in the United States. Employment in the field is expected to grow faster than the average for all careers through 2018.

FAST FACTS

High School Subjects
Biology
Mathematics

Personal Skills
Helping
Technical

Minimum Education Level
Some postsecondary training

Salary Range
$35,000 to $61,000 to $107,000+

Employment Outlook
Faster than the average

O*NET-SOC
29-1124.00, 29-2032.00,
29-2033.00, 29-2034.00,
29-2034.01, 29-2034.02

GOE
14.05.01

DOT
078

NOC
3215

THE JOB

Radiologic technicians and technologists operate and maintain diagnostic imaging equipment and provide radiologists with detailed images used in the diagnosis and treatment of patients. Before starting a procedure, technicians and technologists first prepare the examining room. They make sure equipment is in working condition and ready for use and that all sterile and non-sterile supplies, including contrast materials, catheters, film, and chemicals, needed for the procedure are available. Equipment and supplies are determined by the types of images ordered by the physician.

When the patient arrives, technicians and technologists take a brief medical history, explain the procedure, and answer any questions the patient may have. Then they position the patient in order to achieve the best angle for exposure. They angle or adjust the height of instruments to concentrate on a particular area of the body. They use measuring sticks or tapes to gauge the thickness of the area to be imaged. Patients are draped with lead aprons or shields as a protective measure against radiation exposure. Technicians and technologists place x-ray film under the area, then expose and develop the film using film processors or computer-generated methods.

Technicians and technologists produce x-rays of proper density, detail, or contrast as presented in the physician's orders. They repeat exposures as needed, rejecting any work that does not meet established requirements or standards.

Radiologic technologists complete advanced training in order to operate and maintain equipment that produces more specialized images. They often specialize in one or more diagnostic procedures. The following paragraphs detail these specialties.

Bone densitometry technologists use special x-ray equipment to measure bone mineral density. Usual sites for this procedure include the wrist, spine, heel, or hip. Physicians use this information to determine if patients have or are at risk for osteoporosis, to track general bone loss, or for other reasons.

Cardiovascular-interventional technologists use biplane fluoroscopy and other techniques to guide small instruments, such as catheters, vena cava filters, or stents during interventional or therapeutic procedures. Examples of some procedures are angioplasty, embolizations, and biopsies, all minimally invasive treatments done to cure or alleviate symptoms of vascular disease, stroke, or cancer.

Computed tomography (CT) technologists use x-ray equipment that rotates around the patient during the imaging procedure to obtain cross sections, or slices, of a particular part of the body. Using a computer, these slices are stacked together, creating a three-dimensional image. Since the complete image allows a view of an organ's interior, physicians may order a CT to rule out possible brain hemorrhages or appendicitis, among other diseases and conditions.

Diagnostic medical sonographers use ultrasound equipment to obtain images of organs, tissues, and blood vessels in the body, or in the case of pregnancy, to assess the health and development of a fetus. This technology is increasingly being used to detect heart attacks and heart and vascular disease. Using a transducer or monitor held to a particular area of the patient's body, the sonographer records echoes of high-frequency sound waves as they bounce from the patient's organs, her tissues, or the fetus back to the equipment. These echoes are recorded electronically and generated into a real-time image and recorded for later review by physicians. Sonographers use their knowledge of sonographic technology and the human body to determine if the images they have recorded are sufficient for analysis by a physician, or if more comprehensive tests are necessary. Specialties in the field include abdominal, breast, echocardiography, neurosonography, obstetrics/gynecology, ophthalmology, pediatric echocardiography, and peripheral vascular doppler.

Magnetic resonance imaging technologists operate machinery that uses strong magnetic fields or radio frequency waves to image body tissues.

These signals are measured by a computer and processed into a detailed three-dimensional image of a particular part of the patient's body. MRIs are often ordered to identify the extent of injury to the ligaments or locate tumors in the brain.

Mammographers operate special low-dose x-ray equipment that produces images of the breast. They complete comprehensive education and training, as mandated by federal law, namely the Mammography Quality Standards Act.

Nuclear medicine is used to diagnose, manage, treat, and prevent diseases. *Nuclear medicine technologists* use small amounts of radioactive materials, or radiopharmaceuticals, to obtain information about organs, tissues, or bones, and their degree of health. According to the American Society of Radiologic Technologists, common nuclear medicine applications include "diagnosis and treatment of hyperthyroidism (Graves' Disease), cardiac stress tests to analyze heart function, bone scans for orthopedic injuries, lung scans for blood clots, and liver and gall bladder procedures to diagnose abnormal functions or blockages." Nuclear medicine technologists prepare radiopharmaceutical solutions for patients to drink; once ingested, these images allow special cameras to create an image of a particular organ, bone, or tissue area. These solutions may also be administered by injection or other methods.

Some technologists, after additional training and much experience, work as part of the radiation oncology team. They help radiation oncologists, medical physicists, and nurses diagnose and treat many different types of cancers. *Medical dosimetrists* calculate and measure the dose of radiation delivered to the site of a tumor, using treatment plans developed by an oncologist. They use three-dimensional computer models to determine how and where to deliver the radiation. Before treatment begins, the dosimetrist runs computer simulations to ensure that his or her treatment plan will work as envisioned. Then the dosimetrist instructs the *radiation therapist* to deliver the radiation. Other duties for dosimetrists include documenting treatment plans, calibrating radiation oncology equipment, conducting research, and teaching medical dosimetry students at colleges and universities. Radiation therapists, using treatment plans developed by a radiation oncologist and medical dosimetrist, dispense targeted radiation doses to the patient's body. Repeated exposure to radiation doses often shrinks and destroys malignant sites or cancerous cells. Treatment duration varies for cancer patients, but it typically lasts three to five days a week for four to seven weeks.

Depending on the size of the office or practice, radiologic technicians and technologists may have additional duties including calling for equipment maintenance when needed, ordering additional supplies, scheduling work shifts, and handling other administrative duties.

Full-time radiologic technologists and technicians work about 40 hours a week. Some technologists and technicians work during the evenings, on weekends, and some may be on call to accommodate patients' needs. This job can be physically demanding, as technologists and technicians are on their feet for most of the day. While most procedures are done in examining rooms, some are conducted at the patient's bedside using portable imaging equipment. Some travel is also required when working with home health patients. In these cases, portable diagnostic equipment is usually transported in vans or other large vehicles to the patient's home.

Radiologic technicians and technologists face an enhanced risk of exposure to radiation. Technologists and technicians wear protective lead aprons, gloves, and other shielding devices to minimize this hazard. Their work stations are located behind protective glass windows or doors to help alleviate exposure. Technicians and technologists wear badges that measure radiation levels in the radiation area, as well as keep detailed records on their cumulative lifetime exposure to radiation.

REQUIREMENTS

HIGH SCHOOL

In high school, take physics, algebra, anatomy and physiology, science, chemistry, and biology courses. Classes in English and speech will help you develop your communication skills, and computer science courses will help you become adept at using computers and software programs.

POSTSECONDARY TRAINING

Educational requirements vary by specialty, but radiologic technicians and technologists typically require education ranging from a certificate to a bachelor's degree to enter the field. The associate's degree is the most common educational award for technicians and technologists.

Radiography, magnetic resonance, medical dosimetry, and radiation therapy educational programs are accredited by the Joint Review Committee on Education in Radiologic Technology (www.jrcert.org/cert/Search.jsp). The Joint Review Committee on Education in Diagnostic Medical Sonography (www.jrcdms.org) and the Commission on Accreditation of Allied Health Education Programs (www.caahep.org/Find-An-Accredited-Program) accredit programs in diagnostic medical sonography. The Joint Review Committee on Education Programs in Nuclear Medicine Technology (www.jrcnmt.org/acprograms.asp) accredits nuclear medicine technology educational programs.

CERTIFICATION AND LICENSING

The American Registry of Radiologic Technologists (ARRT, www.arrt.org) offers certification to those who have graduated from an ARRT-approved program and pass an examination. The American Registry for Diagnostic Medical Sonography (www.ardms.org), the ARRT, and Cardiovascular Credentialing International (www.cci-online.org) offer certification to diagnostic medical sonographers. Certification for nuclear medicine technologists is offered by the ARRT and the Nuclear Medicine Technology Certification Board (www.nmtcb.org). The Medical Dosimetrist Certification Board (www.mdcb.org) awards certification to dosimetrists. Certification, while voluntary, is highly recommended. It is an excellent way to stand out from other job applicants and demonstrate your abilities to prospective employers.

Most states require radiologic technicians and technologists to be licensed. Licensing requirements vary by state and specialty. Contact your state's department of regulation for information on requirements in your state.

OTHER REQUIREMENTS

To be a successful radiologic technician or technologist, you should have excellent hand-eye coordination in order to effectively operate equipment and create quality images; physical stamina, since you will be on your feet for long periods of time and be required to turn and lift patients; and good communication skills because you will have to carefully explain procedures to patients and interact closely with doctors and other medical professionals to understand imaging procedures and treatment goals. You should also have compassion and empathy because you will often work with sick and sometimes scared or angry patients who need encouragement as they face health challenges. Other important traits for technicians and technologists include strong observation skills, an analytical mind, proficiency with computers and technology, and a willingness to continue to learn throughout your career.

EXPLORING

There are many ways to learn more about a career as a radiologic technician or technologist. You can read books and journals (such as *Radiologic Technology* and *Radiation Therapist*, www.asrt.org/content/Publications/_asrtpublications.aspx) about the field and visit the websites of college radiology educational programs to learn about typical classes and possible career paths. Ask your teacher or school counselor to arrange an information interview with a radiologic technician or technologist. Professional associations can also provide information about the field. The American Society of Radiologic Technologists offers information on education and careers at its website, www.asrt.org. Many other associations are listed in the For More Information section of this article. You should also try to land a part-time job in a medical office that employs radiologic technicians and technologists. This will give you a chance to interact with workers in the field and see if the career is a good fit for your interests and abilities.

EMPLOYERS

Approximately 286,800 radiologic technicians and technologists are employed in the United States. Hospitals employ 61 percent of technicians and technologists. Other employers include clinics, medical and diagnostic laboratories, offices of physicians, outpatient care centers, cancer care facilities, and other health care facilities.

GETTING A JOB

Many radiologic technicians and technologists obtain their first jobs as a result of contacts made through college internships, career fairs, or networking events. Others seek assistance in obtaining job leads from college career services offices, newspaper want ads, and employment websites. Additionally, professional associations, such as the the American Society of Radiologic Technologists, the American Institute of Ultrasound in Medicine, the Society for Nuclear Medicine, and the American Society of Echocardiography, provide job listings at their websites. See For More Information for contact information for these and other organizations. Those interested in positions with the federal government should visit the U.S. Office of Personnel Management's website, www.usajobs.opm.gov.

ADVANCEMENT

General radiologic technicians and technologists with experience and additional educational training can become specialists in bone densitometry, mammography, magnetic resonance imaging, and other specialties. The typical managerial track for technicians and technologists is promotion to supervisor, chief radiologic technologist, and department administrator or director. Radiology department directors may require the completion of classes or a master's degree in business or health administration. Other possibilities include working as sales representatives and college educators.

EARNINGS

Salaries for radiologic technologists and technicians vary by type of employer, geographic region, and the worker's experience, education, and skill level. Median annual salaries for radiologic technologists and technicians were $61,733 in 2010, according to the American Society of Radiologic Technologists.

Salaries for radiologic technicians and technologists ranged from less than $35,700 to $75,440 or more in 2009, according to the U.S. Department of Labor (USDL). The USDL reports the following mean annual earnings for radiologic technologists and technicians by employer: medical and diagnostic laboratories, $57,250; federal government, $56,140; general medical and surgical hospitals, $54,770; outpatient care centers, $52,950; and offices of physicians, $50,860.

In 2009, salaries for nuclear medicine technologists ranged from less than $48,710 to $90,650 or more, according to the USDL. They had median annual earnings of $67,910.

Diagnostic medical sonographers earned median annual salaries of $63,010 in 2009, according to the USDL. Ten percent earned less than $43,990, and 10 percent earned $85,950 or more.

Radiation therapists earned salaries that ranged from less than $49,980 to $107,230 or more in 2009, according to the USDL. They had median annual earnings of $74,170.

Employers offer a variety of benefits, including the following: medical, dental, and life insurance; paid holidays, vacations, and sick and personal days; 401(k) plans; profit-sharing plans; retirement and pension plans; and educational-assistance programs. Part-time workers must provide their own benefits.

EMPLOYMENT OUTLOOK

Employment in the field is expected to grow faster than the average for all careers through 2018, according to the U.S. Department of Labor. Demand will increase as the U.S. population grows and ages, creating a need for more diagnostic procedures. In addition, radiation technology has become safer in recent years, and more procedures are being done—especially to detect diseases earlier and to reduce health care insurance costs. Technicians and technologists who are skilled in more than one imaging modality—such as magnetic resonance imaging (MRI) and computed tomography (CT)—will have the best job prospects. In fact, MRI and CT technologists and technicians will be in especially strong demand in coming years due to the accuracy of these imaging technologies. Workers who are willing to relocate to areas of the United States that are experiencing shortages of workers will also have strong employment prospects. (The recent recession in the United States has created a challenging job market

Employment Growth in the Health Care Industry by Employment Sector, 2008-18

Home Healthcare Services: +46.1 percent

Offices of Other Health Practitioners: +41.3 percent

Medical and Diagnostic Laboratories: +39.8 percent

Outpatient Care Centers: +38.6 percent

Offices of Physicians: +34.1 percent

Offices of Dentists: +28.5 percent

Nursing and Residential Care Facilities: +21.2 percent

Source: U.S. Department of Labor

for radiologic technology professionals. Sal Martino, chief executive officer of the American Society of Radiologic Technologists, offers a more sober assessment of the current market. See his interview on pages 188-189 for his views on the current and future employment outlook for radiologic technicians and technologists.)

Nuclear medicine technologists should expect strong competition for jobs. Although nuclear medicine technology is increasingly being used to diagnose, manage, treat, and prevent diseases, there are more technologists than available positions.

FOR MORE INFORMATION

Contact the following organizations for more information on education, careers, and certification.

**Alliance of
Cardiovascular Professionals**
PO Box 2007
Midlothian, VA 23113-9007
www.acp-online.org

**American Association
of Medical Dosimetrists**
12100 Sunset Hills Road, Suite 130
Reston, VA 20190-3221
aamd@medicaldosimetry.org
www.medicaldosimetry.org

**American Institute of
Ultrasound in Medicine**
14750 Sweitzer Lane, Suite 100
Laurel, MD 20707-5906
www.aium.org

**American Society
for Radiation Oncology**
8280 Willow Oaks Corporate Drive,
Suite 500
Fairfax, VA 22031-4514
www.astro.org

**American Society of
Echocardiography**
2100 Gateway Centre Boulevard,
Suite 310
Morrisville, NC 27560-6230
www.asecho.org

**American Society
of Radiologic Technologists**
15000 Central Avenue, SE
Albuquerque, NM 87123-3909
customerinfo@asrt.org
www.asrt.org

**Association of Vascular and
Interventional Radiographers**
12100 Sunset Hills Road, Suite 130
Reston, VA 20190-3221
www.avir.org

**International Society
for Clinical Densitometry**
306 Industrial Park Road, Suite 208
Middletown, CT 06457-7557
iscd@iscd.org
www.iscd.org

**International Society for
Magnetic Resonance in Medicine**
2030 Addison Street, 7th Floor
Berkeley, CA 94704-1158
510-841-1899
www.ismrm.org

**Society for Cardiovascular
Magnetic Resonance**
19 Mantua Road
Mt. Royal, NJ 08061-1006
hq@scmr.org
www.scmr.org

Society for Nuclear Medicine
1850 Samuel Morse Drive
Reston, VA 20190-5316
703-708-9000
www.snm.org

Society for Vascular Ultrasound
4601 Presidents Drive, Suite 260
Lanham, MD 20706-4831
301-459-7550
svuinfo@svunet.org
www.svunet.org

**Society of Diagnostic
Medical Sonography**
2745 Dallas Parkway, Suite 350
Plano, TX 75093-8730
800-229-9506
www.sdms.org

For information on educational training and careers in Canada, contact
**Canadian Association of Medical
Radiation Technologists**
1000-85 Albert Street
Ottawa, ON K1P 6A4 Canada
613-234-0012
www.camrt.ca

Interview: Sal Martino

Sal Martino, Ed.D., R.T., FASRT, CAE is the chief executive officer of the American Society of Radiologic Technologists (ASRT). He discussed the field of medical imaging with the editors of *Hot Health Care Careers*.

Q. **What is one thing that young people may not know about a career in medical imaging and radiation therapy?**

A. Radiologic technologists should possess excellent patient care skills. It's not uncommon for prospective students to become enamored with the technology related to medical imaging and radiation therapy and forget that radiologic technologists work hard every day to improve patient outcomes. Although the profession is extremely high-tech and exciting, it is the human side of the radiologic science profession that is most significant. A technologist who has a great deal of technical expertise will not provide the best overall examination for a patient if he or she fails to include the human touch.

Q. **What advice would you offer radiologic technology students as they graduate and look for jobs?**

A. As most of your readers are probably aware, the job market is tight in all areas right now, and the radiologic technology field is no exception. That being said, there are some jobs out there if a graduate is willing to relocate or work during off-hours. The most important step graduates can take right now is to get a foot in the door at a health care institution. The job may not be the desired shift or location, but it may lead to increased opportunities as radiologic technologists retire and the field expands in the future. In addition, this is a wonderful time for graduates to expand their skill sets and prepare themselves for the future. Advancements in computed tomography, magnetic resonance, imaging informatics, and many other modalities offer exciting professional opportunities in the future for those technologists who take the initiative to learn about different modalities and specialty areas.

Q. **What is the employment outlook for medical imaging and radiation therapy professionals? How is the field changing, and what are the most promising career paths in the field?**

A. Right now the medical imaging community seems to be holding its breath. Changes in health care, a sluggish economy, and an unknown future have resulted in a tighter job market. This outlook is not unique to medical imaging; many professions have seen a tightening in the job market in recent years. In medical imaging we have seen a large shortage evaporate in just five or six years. We don't know if another shortage of medical imaging technologists will occur once the economy stabilizes and many health care questions are answered. The ASRT has conducted a great deal of research in the past that shows the demand for radiologic technologists increasing and decreasing. Right now we are in a period of decreased demand, but these periods are generally followed by a demand surge.

Q. Can you tell us about the American Society of Radiologic Technologists? How important is membership in the ASRT for career success?

A. The American Society of Radiologic Technologists represents health care professionals who perform medical imaging examinations or deliver radiation therapy. The ASRT's role is to ensure that its 138,000 members keep up with the technological advances, regulatory changes, and economic forces that are transforming their profession. ASRT's educational resources, career development tools, practice standards, and advocacy efforts help radiologic technologists improve the quality of patient care. It is the leading provider of continuing education in the radiologic sciences and the principal source for research data on the profession.

The ASRT provides its members with a variety of opportunities to strengthen their skills and advance their careers. Whether keeping up to date with the latest professional news or staying ahead with continuing education, ASRT members have access to the information they need to succeed. There is no better investment a radiologic technologist can make than being a member of the ASRT.

Interview: Mark Daniels

Mark Daniels, B.S., RT, CMD is a medical dosimetrist at Virginia Mason Medical Center in Seattle, Washington, and the educational coordinator of the Medical Dosimetry Program (http://bellevuecollege.edu/health/imaging/dosimetry.asp) at Bellevue College. He discussed his career and the field of medical dosimetry with the editors of *Hot Health Care Careers*.

Q. What is one thing that young people may not know about a career in medical dosimetry?

A. When I was in high school, I recall taking trigonometry and thinking to myself: "When will I EVER use this in 'real life'?" Well, here it is...but it is different than just "doing math." As a member of the radiation oncology team (radiation oncology is the use of controlled radiation to treat patients with cancer and some select benign conditions), medical dosimetry is specialized in that dosimetrists apply both complex mathematical and physics-based principles to the betterment of care for individuals. A mentor of mine once told me that medical dosimetry is the perfect marriage between science and art, and I have never seen anything but 100 percent truth in that statement. Dosimetrists use creative methods to achieve a desired plan, shaping and carving radiation doses around portions of a patient's body that don't need radiation and delivering the dose to the areas that do. And because every patient's body is unique, every plan presents a unique challenge and opportunity to "solve the puzzle" of how to deliver the radiation safely and accurately to the area prescribed.

Q. What are your primary and secondary duties as a medical dosimetrist?

A. As dosimetrists, our primary duties include using sophisticated treatment planning computers and various calculations to create a radiation treatment plan based on a radiation oncologist's prescription. We are responsible for documenting relevant and pertinent information in the patient record, and to independently verify the accuracy of all calculations and plans in tandem with departmental guidelines and under the supervision of the medical physicist. Secondary duties include providing physics support to the medical physicist in the roles of treatment and/or linear accelerator quality assurance. Further, we are often utilized in the role of an educator in facilities that have radiation oncology residents, radiation therapy students, and/or medical dosimetry students.

Q.   What do you like most and least about your career?

A.   What I like the most is the continual technological advancements seen in our field. Complex treatment planning systems employ many utilities that dosimetrists use every day to achieve the desired outcome, and when those utilities are improved through research and development, our ability to target and place the radiation exactly where we need it (and avoid areas where we don't) is enhanced in tandem. Ultimately, the benefit to these advancements is to our patient population, either through improved outcomes or reduced side effects, and that is the most rewarding part of our profession...knowing that what we do makes a difference every day in someone else's life.

What I like the least about the medical dosimetry career is the lack of patient contact. I, as did many others in dosimetry, started out as a radiation therapist. My daily job entailed treating patients with the very plans I now generate as a dosimetrist. Patients often come in for several weeks of therapy, and over time, you develop a rapport and professional relationship that is very rewarding. This is lost at times in medical dosimetry, as the time spent constructing the plans restricts our ability to be in contact with the patients.

Q.   Can you please tell us about your program?

A.   This is an excellent question, as the answer is ever changing. Medical dosimetry itself does not have a uniform path to practice. There are several programs in the nation with degree ranges from a certificate in medical dosimetry (no degree offered) up to and including a master's degree in medical dosimetry. What is used as a benchmark for qualified practice in medical dosimetry is certification through the Medical Dosimetrist Certification Board (MDCB) (national board exam administrators). Currently, there are three routes to certification through the MDCB. Visit www.mdcb.org for more information on these paths.

Q.   What types of students pursue study in your program?

A.   The qualities and characteristics of an ideal dosimetry student would be someone who (1) enjoys working in health care (it is not for everyone); (2) possesses high levels of attention to detail; (3) is comfortable with computers and various operating systems; (4) has a high degree of understanding of mathematics and physics and would be comfortable applying abstract theory and concepts into clinical practice and the "real world"; and, (5) is capable of demonstrating excellent written, verbal, and interpersonal communication skills.

Q. What advice would you offer medical dosimetry students as they graduate and look for jobs?

A. As students graduate and compete for positions, the jobs are ultimately given to the best-qualified candidate. This presents unique difficulties for new graduates, as they do not have much experience; therefore, excelling in school, having solid professional references and a varied clinical experience, and showing self-motivated learning while in their program are all very positive traits that can be expanded on during an interview. One of the biggest things to remember is that experience is worth a small fortune, so being flexible in where a newly graduated student takes that first job in the interest of gaining the experience can pay off huge dividends down the road. As with any job opportunity, evaluating a clinic's strengths and weaknesses is important to see how your skill set matches their clinical needs. Finally, ask yourself about staffing levels in the department's dosimetry and physics areas: can this department help me achieve my personal and professional goals, or will I be left on an island without any help?

Q. What is the employment outlook for medical dosimetrists?

A. The dynamic world of health care is impossible to predict. Job outlook has been historically very healthy for medical dosimetrists, while recent changes show a slight narrowing of openings relative to numbers of students/dosimetrists applying for a given clinical position. Jobs, however, are not always limited to the clinical setting. While not necessarily recommended for newly graduating students, industry jobs are ever present for dosimetrists. There are positions with major corporations that employ dosimetrists in their radiation oncology divisions for applications training and support, research and development of new planning systems/applications, and government relations focused on corporate compliance and technology approval for clinical use. Invariably, there are dosimetry jobs available and, as in many fields, the "premier" center or location may not be available, but a more remote opening might be. One thing I have gleaned from my years in this field is that some of the more remote centers often provide the same level of service and treatment options (if not more) than the competing major academic sites/institutions. So it is not always about the "name" of the clinic where you choose to work as much as the caliber of programs offered by the clinic aligning with your employment goals that can make a new dosimetrist a content professional on the radiation oncology team.

REGISTERED NURSES

OVERVIEW

Registered nurses work to promote health, prevent disease, and help patients who are sick or injured. They also serve as health educators for patients, families, and communities. Registered nurses train for the field by earning a bachelor's degree, an associate degree, or a diploma in nursing from an approved nursing program. Registered nurses who decide to become advanced practice nurses (clinical nurse specialists, nurse anesthetists, nurse-midwives, and nurse practitioners) must earn master's degrees and industry certifications. Registered nurses (RNs) make up the largest occupational group in the health care industry, comprising approximately 2.6 million jobs. Employment opportunities for RNs are expected to be excellent through 2018.

THE JOB

Most RNs provide direct patient care. They observe, assess, and record patient symptoms, reactions, and progress. Nurses collaborate with physicians and other medical professionals on patient care, treatments, and examinations, and they administer medications.

RNs work closely with physicians to care for patients. It is their job to implement the doctor's orders regarding the treatment of a patient. In addition to interacting with patients, RNs also have a lot of contact with patients' families, so they must have good "bedside manner" and put people at ease.

Specific work responsibilities vary from one RN to the next. An RN's duties and title are often determined by his or her work setting, such as *emergency room nurses,* who work in hospital emergency rooms, or *radiology nurses,* who administer x-rays and other body scans to patients or care for those undergoing radiation treatments for cancer. These nurses generally work in hospitals, clinics, or outpatient care facilities. RNs can also work outside of health care facilities, in settings such as schools, workplaces, and summer camps.

Other nurses are defined by the types of patients served. *Hematology nurses,* for example, help patients with blood disorders. *Oncology nurses* specialize in treating patients with cancer. These nurses are employed virtually anywhere, including physicians' offices, outpatient treatment facilities, home health care agencies, and hospitals. Those that specialize in a disease or condition may also specialize in the age of the patients served. Some examples include *neonatal nurses* (newborns), *pediatric nurses* (children and adolescents), and *geriatric nurses* (the elderly).

Finally, other RNs specialize in working with one or more organs or systems, such as *respiratory nurses,* who care for those with respiratory illnesses such as cystic fibrosis or asthma. RNs specializing in treatment of a particular organ or body system usually are employed in hospital specialty or critical care units, specialty clinics, and outpatient care facilities.

RNs can be one or a combination of these nursing types, such as a *geriatric dialysis nurse,* who specializes in care for elderly patients with kidney failure.

Registered nurses who pursue advanced degrees and certification are called *advanced practice nurses (APNs).* There are four advanced practice nursing specialties: *clinical nurse specialists, nurse anesthetists, nurse-midwives,* and *nurse practitioners.* For detailed information on these specialties, see the article, Advanced Practice Nurses, in this book.

Instead of working in teams under the direction of a physician, APNs work relatively independently. Clinical nurse specialists provide specialized expertise in a specific area of nursing, such as rehabilitation, mental health, or geriatrics. Nurse anesthetists administer anesthesia and provide pain management services before and after surgical, therapeutic, diagnostic, and obstetric procedures. Nurse-midwives provide primary care to women, including gynecological exams, prenatal and neonatal care, and direct assistance in labor and delivery. Finally, nurse practitioners serve as primary and specialty care providers, providing a blend of nursing and health care services to patients and families. Specialties include pediatrics, family practice, and women's health, among others.

In addition to caring for patients with existing conditions and illnesses, nurses also perform a valuable service by providing education and preventive care to healthy populations. A good example of this type of nurse includes an *occupational health nurse,* who seeks to prevent job-related injuries and illnesses and supports employers in implementing health and safety standards.

Some RNs work in applied nursing jobs, or positions that require the medical knowledge of a nurse without the traditional hands-on work with patients. The following paragraphs detail some popular applied nursing specialties:

Nurse educators evaluate existing or create new professional development plans for student nurses and RNs. They teach a variety of nursing classes to students.

Forensic nurses provide legal testimony in investigations of accidents or crimes.

Legal nurse consultants are registered nurses with considerable nursing experience and knowledge of the legal system. They use these skills to assist lawyers in health-care-related cases. According to the American Association of Legal Nurse Consultants (www.aalnc.org), legal nurse consultants offer support to the law profession in the following practice areas: personal injury, product liability, medical malpractice, workers' compensation, toxic torts, risk management, medical licensure investigation, criminal law, elder law, and fraud and abuse compliance.

Nursing informatics specialists organize a database of patients' medical information in an accessible format. They may customize and test the database according to the needs of different medical departments or specialties. Nursing informatics specialists also train nurses on computer charting, which consists of adding information to or retrieving it from the database. They may also write and install new programs or software applications to help nursing staffs work more efficiently.

As the types of nursing varieties are numerous, so are the settings in which nurses work. In addition to hospitals, doctor's offices, and medical clinics, nurses work in patients' homes, schools, large corporations, community centers, and other locations. Hospitals or other 24-hour facilities must be staffed around the clock, so some nurses work holidays, weekends, and overnight shifts.

Nurses follow strict guidelines in handling hazardous medical waste or dangerous instruments such as needles. They are also exposed to patients with contagious diseases, so they must wear protective gear such as masks and gloves. Hand washing is constant and methodical in nursing to prevent the transmission of communicable diseases.

While their jobs may be stressful, most nurses find caring for others enjoyable and rewarding.

REQUIREMENTS

HIGH SCHOOL

Take health, mathematics, biology, anatomy and physiology, chemistry, physics, English, speech, and computer science classes in high school to prepare for a career in nursing.

POSTSECONDARY TRAINING

Prospective RNs have the option of pursuing one of three training paths: associate's degree, diploma, and bachelor's degree. Associate's degree programs in nursing last two years and are offered by community colleges. Diploma programs in nursing typically last three years and are offered by hospitals and independent schools. Bachelor of science in nursing programs are offered by colleges and universities. They typically take four—and sometimes five—years to complete. Graduates of all three paths are known as graduate nurses and must take a licensing exam in their state to obtain the RN designation. Visit www.discovernursing.com for a database of nursing programs.

Students who are interested in becoming nurse managers should earn at least a bachelor's degree. Those interested in becoming nursing educators, advanced practice nurses, or advancing as an RN should earn at least a master's degree in nursing, plus industry certifications.

CERTIFICATION AND LICENSING

Certification or credentialing, while voluntary, is highly recommended. It is an excellent way to stand out from other job applicants and demonstrate your abilities to prospective employers. Certification is offered by the American Nursing Credentialing Center, the National League for Nursing, and many other nursing organizations.

Nurses must be licensed to practice nursing in all states and the District of Columbia. Licensure requirements vary by state but typically include graduating from an approved nursing school and passing the National Council Licensure Examination, which is administered by the National Council of State Boards of Nursing.

OTHER REQUIREMENTS

To be a successful registered nurse, you should be detail oriented, have excellent communication skills, be sympathetic and caring, be calm under pressure, have leadership skills, and be willing to continue to learn throughout your career. You will need to be emotionally strong, since you will encounter many heartbreaking cases and emergency situations. You will also need to be physically fit, since you will spend many hours on your feet and often bend and stoop, and lift patients, as needed.

EXPLORING

Read books about nursing, talk with your counselor or teacher about setting up a presentation by a nurse, take a tour of a hospital or other health care setting, or volunteer at one of these facilities. Nursing websites, including those of professional associations, can also be a good source of information. Here are a few suggestions: Cybernurse.com (www.cybernurse.com), Discover Nursing (www.discovernursing.com), Nurse.com (www.nurse.com), and

Books to Read

Catalano, Joseph T. *Nursing Now: Today's Issues, Tomorrow's Trends.* 5th ed. Philadelphia: F. A. Davis Company, 2008.

Novotny, Jeanne M., Doris T. Lippman, Nicole K. Sanders, and Joyce J. Fitzpatrick. *101 Careers in Nursing.* New York: Springer Publishing Company, 2006.

Peterson, Veronica. *Just the Facts: A Pocket Guide to Nursing.* 4th ed. St. Louis: Mosby, 2008.

Potter, Patricia A., and Anne Griffin Perry. *Fundamentals of Nursing.* 6th ed. St. Louis: Mosby, 2008.

Vallano, Annette. *Your Career In Nursing: Manage Your Future in the Changing World of Healthcare.* 5th ed. New York: Kaplan Publishing, 2008.

Futures in Nursing (http://futuresinnursing.org). You should also join Future Nurses organizations or student health clubs at your school.

EMPLOYERS

Approximately 2.6 million registered nurses are employed in the United States. The U.S. Department of Labor reports that 60 percent of registered nurses work at hospitals, 8 percent in offices of physicians, 5 percent in home health care services, 5 percent in nursing care facilities, and 3 percent in employment services. Other RNs are employed by colleges and universities, prisons, corporations, government agencies, and social assistance agencies. Some RNs with advanced education work as college nursing professors.

GETTING A JOB

Many registered nurses obtain their first jobs as a result of contacts made through college internships, clinical rotations, or networking events. Others seek assistance in obtaining job leads from college career services offices, newspaper want ads, and employment websites. Additionally, professional associations, such as the American Nurses Association, provide job listings at their websites. See For More Information for a list of organizations. Those interested in positions with the federal government should visit the U.S. Office of Personnel Management's website, www.usajobs.opm.gov.

ADVANCEMENT

There are many advancement opportunities for registered nurses. Those who start their careers as staff nurses can become nurse managers or head nurses. Those already in management positions can advance from assistant unit manager or head nurse to more senior-level administrative roles such as assistant director, director, vice president, or chief of nursing. Registered nurses can earn a master's degree and industry certifications and become advanced practice nurses. Some nurses become college professors. Others work in research or serve as consultants for insurance companies, pharmaceutical manufacturers, and law firms.

EARNINGS

Median annual salaries for registered nurses were $63,750 in 2009, according to the U.S. Department of Labor (USDL). Salaries ranged from less than $43,970 to $93,700 or more. The USDL reports the following mean annual earnings for registered nurses by employer: federal government, $77,830; general medical and surgical hospitals, $67,740; offices of physicians, $67,290; outpatient care centers, $65,690; home health care services, $63,300; and nursing care facilities, $59,320.

Employers offer a variety of benefits, including the following: medical, dental, and life insurance; paid holidays, vacations, and sick days; personal days; 401(k) plans; profit-sharing plans; retirement and pension plans; and educational assistance programs. Self-employed workers must provide their own benefits.

EMPLOYMENT OUTLOOK

The career outlook for nurses is excellent. The U.S. Department of Labor (USDL) predicts that more than 737,000 new and replacement nurses will be needed by 2018 to care for the growing—and aging—U.S. population. The next several years will be an excellent time to pursue a career in nursing. Employment for nurses will be best in offices of physicians. This sector will experience growth of 48 percent through 2018, according to the USDL. Employment for nurses in home health care services will grow by 33 percent; by 25 percent in nursing care facilities; by 24 percent in employment services; and by 17 percent in hospitals, public and private.

Many nursing specialties are experiencing strong growth. One of the fastest-growing areas is the care of geriatric populations. As baby boomers continue to reach their mid-60s and beyond, there will be increasing demand for nurses with specialized training in geriatric care. According to *Who Will Care for Each of Us?: America's Coming Health Care Crisis*, the ratio of potential caregivers to those who need care (including the growing elderly population) will decrease by 40 percent between 2010 and 2030, creating a strong need for health care professionals, including nurses. In addition, the USDL reports that clinical nurse specialists, nurse practitioners, nurse-midwives, and nurse anesthetists will be in strong demand. Opportunities should also be good for nurses who "provide specialized long-term rehabilitation for stroke and head injury patients."

Despite the rosy outlook, the American Association of Colleges of Nursing (AACN) reports that enrollment in entry-level baccalaureate nursing programs grew by only 3.6 percent from 2008 to 2009. This growth is not enough to fill all available openings. The Health Resources and Services Administration states that "to meet the projected growth in demand for RN services, the U.S. must graduate approximately 90 percent more nurses from U.S. nursing programs."

Many students are interested in studying nursing, but they are finding it hard to land a coveted spot in nursing school. The AACN notes that 39,423 qualified applicants to baccalaureate and graduate nursing programs were turned away in 2009 due to "insufficient number of faculty, clinical sites, classroom space, clinical preceptors, and budget constraints."

What is causing the faculty shortages? Earnings and age are two of the most significant factors. According to the *New York Times,* nursing educators earn 40 to 50 percent less than nurses employed in clinical settings, which keeps qualified nurses who might be interested in pursuing a career in academe on the sidelines due to financial considerations. Additionally, many nurses are becoming educators late in their careers—the average age of nursing educators is 57—and many educators are retiring without being replaced.

To address these shortages, professional nursing organizations are working to secure federal funding for faculty development programs, creating scholarship programs for doctoral education (the typical educational requirement for top positions in nursing education), and attempting to develop a more direct route to the Ph.D. in order to encourage students to pursue nursing education at a younger age.

FOR MORE INFORMATION

The following organizations provide a wealth of resources and information related to registered nursing. For a list of advanced practice nursing associations, see the For More Information section of the Advanced Practice Nurses article in this book.

For information on opportunities for men in nursing, contact
**American Assembly
for Men in Nursing**
PO Box 130220
Birmingham, AL 35213-0220
www.aamn.org

For information on careers in assisted living facilities, contact
**American Assisted
Living Nurses Association**
PO Box 10469
Napa, CA 94581-2469
www.alnursing.org

For information on accredited nursing programs, contact
**American Association
of Colleges of Nursing**
One Dupont Circle, NW, Suite 530
Washington, DC 20036-1135
www.aacn.nche.edu

The ANA is the largest nursing organization in the United States. Visit its website for a wealth of information about education, careers, and credentialing.
American Nurses Association (ANA)
8515 Georgia Avenue, Suite 400
Silver Spring, MD 20910-3492
www.nursingworld.org

For certification information, contact
**American Nurses
Credentialing Center**
c/o American Nurses Association
8515 Georgia Avenue, Suite 400
Silver Spring, MD 20910-3492
800-284-2378
www.nursecredentialing.org

For industry news, visit the society's website.
**American Society
of Registered Nurses**
1001 Bridgeway, Suite 233
Sausalito, CA 94965-2104
www.asrn.org

For information on licensing, contact
**National Council of
State Boards of Nursing**
111 East Wacker Drive, Suite 2900
Chicago, IL 60601-4277
www.ncsbn.org

For general information about nursing, contact
National League for Nursing
61 Broadway, 33rd Floor
New York, NY 10006-2701
www.nln.org

The N-OADN serves as an advocate for registered nurses who have earned an associate degree. Visit its website for more information.
**National Organization for Associate
Degree Nursing (N-OADN)**
7794 Grow Drive
Pensacola, FL 32514-7072
www.noadn.org

For information on membership, contact
**National Student
Nurses' Association**
45 Main Street, Suite 606
Brooklyn, NY 11201-1099
nsna@nsna.org
www.nsna.org

For resources for aspiring and current nurses with disabilities, visit
ExceptionalNurse.com
www.exceptionalnurse.com

Interview: Thara Gagni

Thara Gagni is a registered nurse in the Medical Intensive Care Unit at Northwestern Memorial Hospital in Chicago, Illinois. She discussed her career with the editors of *Hot Health Care Careers*.

Q. What made you want to enter this career?

A. I entered this career because I always knew that I wanted to be in the medical field. It was not until my freshmen year of college that I narrowed my choice to nursing. My reasons were really quite simple: I enjoyed providing bedside care; I appreciated being able to build personal relationships with my patients and their families; as a nurse I appreciated the focus on taking care of and being the advocate of the patient (whereas I felt doctors took care of the disease); and there was plenty of directions a career in nursing could take.

Q. What is one thing that young people may not know about a career in nursing?

A. There are so many directions a career in nursing can take you. Some people enjoy bedside nursing, but you can go into politics, law, even business with a career in nursing. Our profession is needed literally EVERYWHERE in the world, so whether you're looking for jobs or volunteer opportunities, all you have to do is seek out where and what you want to be with your degree in nursing. The world is truly your oyster.

Q. What are the most important qualities for people in your career?

A. The most personal qualities for people in nursing, in my opinion, are understanding and compassion. If you take time to put yourself in your patient's shoes, or that of his or her family, you show more compassion. Compassion in nursing will always be an important quality, because when you show it and work with it, you provide the best care for your patients.

Professional qualities that are important in nursing are accountability, advocacy, cultural awareness, and flexibility. Nurses need to be aware they will be held accountable for their practice and the care they provide their patients. We deal with peoples' lives, and so being an advocate for our patients, their health and safety, is always a priority. We deal with many cultures and people of different backgrounds; it is important for nurses to be aware that our care may affect them culturally and vice versa. Being sensitive to a patient's culture and background is always important when trying to holistically care for their needs. In nursing, there is constant research, which means new practices, regulations, and evidence-based practice are always emerging. As nurses, we need to be flexible in this evolving profession.

Q. What do you like most and least about your career?

A. I am gratified after making connections with people despite what their admitting diagnosis may have been. I learn so much from their life experiences. And just when you think you've just had it sometimes in this profession, there will always be one family/patient that expresses their sincerest gratitude and appreciation for you and the work you have done. Now THAT makes anything and everything you go through worth it.

What I like the least? Being told that "you are just the nurse." And yes, it happens and it is said more often than you would like to admit.

Q.   What advice would you give to aspiring nurses?

A.   GO FOR IT! The opportunities are truly endless, and there is always room for improvement and advancement in this field. It is a gratifying profession and all that you do will always be of a great service to the rest of the community...and if you want, to the rest of the world.

Q.   What is the employment outlook for registered nurses?

A.   Due to the recent decline of our economy, job opportunities are not as easy to come by. But in all honesty, I truly believe that there will never come a time when nurses are not needed. They will always be a crucial part of the health care system; it is just a matter of initially finding your first experiences and from there discovering your true niche in the nursing profession.

Other Nursing Careers

✔ Camp Nurses

✔ Community Health Nurses

✔ Correctional Facility Nurses

✔ Critical Care Nurses

✔ Gastroenterology Nurses

✔ Health Policy Experts

✔ Hospice Nurses

✔ Labor and Delivery Nurses

✔ Nephrology Nurses

✔ Nurse Attorneys

✔ Nurse Entrepreneurs

✔ Nurse Researchers

✔ Nursing Historians

✔ Nursing Writers

✔ Ophthlamic Nurses

✔ Orthopaedic Nurses

✔ Plastic Surgery Nurses

✔ Poison Information Specialists

✔ Psychiatric Nurses

✔ Rehabilitation Nurses

✔ Reproductive Nurses

✔ Rheumatology Nurses

✔ School Nurses

✔ Substance Abuse Nurses

✔ Transcultural Nurses

✔ Wound and Ostomy Nurses

REHABILITATION COUNSELORS

OVERVIEW

Rehabilitation counselors help people living with disabilities deal with any associated personal, social, or employment effects. They work with people with both physical and emotional disabilities resulting from birth defects, illness, accidents, or other causes. Rehabilitation counselors collaborate with the individual's families or loved ones, physicians, psychologists, employers, and physical therapists to determine the client's strengths and weaknesses and develop a rehabilitation plan for their client. They arrange training to help clients develop job or life skills or even help them find a job. Their main goal is to help their clients live happy and independent lives. You will need a master's degree in rehabilitation counseling or a related field to become a rehabilitation counselor. Approximately 129,500 rehabilitation counselors are employed in the United States. Employment in the field is expected to grow faster than the average for all careers through 2018.

FAST FACTS

High School Subjects
Psychology
Sociology

Personal Skills
Communication
Helping
Technical

Minimum Education Level
Master's degree

Salary Range
$20,000 to $31,000 to $55,000+

Employment Outlook
Faster than the average

O*NET-SOC
21-1015.00

GOE
12.02.02

DOT
045

NOC
4153

THE JOB

Rehabilitation counselors help people with many different kinds of disabilities, including cognitive or learning limitations, psychological conflicts, and physical or functional disabilities. Many times these disabilities are caused by injuries, accidents, birth defects, stress, trauma caused by crime or war, or the process of aging. Rehabilitation counselors work with clients on a one-on-one basis or as part of group counseling. They teach patients how to cope with the challenges of everyday life, find and succeed in a job, or bridge gaps with family and friends, with the ultimate goal of having clients live independent and meaningful lives.

When working with a new client, rehabilitation counselors begin by conducting a complete assessment of the individual. They evaluate the patient's strengths and identify any weaknesses or limitations. For example, if working with a client who has Down syndrome, rehabilitation counselors will take into account any cognitive or learning disabilities, as well as any physical limitations, which could hamper employment opportunities. They may suggest personal and vocational counseling such as physical therapy programs or training to help their client master certain job skills. Rehabilitation counselors provide constant support in all areas and often schedule reviews to keep up with clients' therapy or training progress. Rehabilitation counselors are on call to provide intervention in crisis situations.

If working with a client who has recently suffered an injury or become disabled, rehabilitation counselors may arrange for medical care or treatment. They often take into account their client's financial situation and can arrange for financial assistance if the client qualifies.

Rehabilitation counselors help clients master basic daily living skills and tasks such as cleaning, self-care and grooming, preparing meals, making a household budget, and shopping. They can also help clients develop skills needed to interact with others in the outside world.

While the client is undergoing counseling or training, rehabilitation counselors can search for possible employment opportunities. Certain organizations, such as Goodwill, offer training and placement opportunities for people with disabilities. The rehabilitation counselor often works with a list of such organizations and can suggest placement.

Rehabilitation counselors also tackle any social or environmental barriers that prohibit people with disabilities from living full lives. These barriers can include prejudice, stereotypes, inaccessible information, inaccessible buildings or transportation, as well as companies with inflexible practices. If not already covered by federal law, rehabilitation counselors fight for accessible walkways and stairs, wider entrance ways or hallways, or even accessible forms of public transportation—practically anything that would help disabled people improve their mobility. If counseling someone with impaired vision, rehabilitation counselors might lobby a company to provide signs in Braille or ask a school to purchase audio versions of textbooks or other materials.

Rehabilitation counselors may also interview the client's family, friends, coworkers, and employer to identify any problems or issues regarding his or her disability. They provide education to help others better understand their client's disability. Oftentimes, rehabilitation counselors can act as a bridge between the client and society.

Rehabilitation counselors spend a great deal of time conferring with the client's family, physician, social workers, and other health care professionals. They often participate in team meetings to discuss the client's progress and make provisions for extra services or training, if needed.

Full-time rehabilitation counselors work 40 hours a week, with some time scheduled in the evenings and on weekends. They work indoors in comfortable, well-lit offices, as well as in the field visiting patients and viewing their work or school environment. A reliable vehicle is usually necessary for travel to and from field sites.

REQUIREMENTS

HIGH SCHOOL

In high school, take courses in psychology, health, computer science, English, and speech.

POSTSECONDARY TRAINING

Some organizations hire rehabilitation counselors with only a bachelor's degree in rehabilitation services, counseling, psychology, sociology, or a human services-related field, but these hires typically work as rehabilitation aides, not as counselors. Most rehabilitation counselors need a master's degree in rehabilitation counseling, general counseling, or counseling psychology to enter the field. Both the Council on Rehabilitation Education and the Council for Accreditation of Counseling and Related Educational Programs accredit counseling educational programs. (See For More Information for contact information for these organizations.) According to the American Medical Association, rehabilitation counselor education programs "typically provide between 18 to 24 months of academic and field-based clinical training. Clinical training consists of a practicum and a minimum of 600 hours of supervised internship experience." Students receive training in counseling theory, skills, and techniques; individual and group counseling; principles of psychiatric rehabilitation; vocational evaluation and work adjustment; career counseling; job development and placement; and other topics.

CERTIFICATION AND LICENSING

Certification and licensing requirements vary greatly based on whether the counselor works for a private or public employer and by state law (although most states have laws requiring counselors to have some form of licensure).

Some counselors choose to become certified by the National Board for Certified Counselors (NBCC). This organization awards a general practice credential of national certified counselor. According to the U.S. Department of Labor, "this national certification is voluntary and is distinct from state licensing. However, in some states, those who pass the national exam are exempt from taking a state certification exam." The NBCC also offers specialty certifications in clinical mental health, addiction, and school counseling.

Voluntary national certification for rehabilitation counselors is available from the Commission on Rehabilitation Counselor Certification. This certification is required by many local and state governments. Contact the Commission for information on certification requirements.

OTHER REQUIREMENTS

Rehabilitation counselors need excellent communication skills, since they spend a great deal of time speaking with patients and their families, lobbying employers, and writing reports. Rehabilitation counselors also confer with physicians, social workers, and therapists regarding the condition and goals of the patient. Successful counselors should be able to work well under pressure, since they may have to deal with the needs of multiple clients at one time. They should also be patient and have a pleasant personality in order to deal with clients who can sometimes be irritable, angry, or depressed. Other important traits for rehabilitation counselors include empathy, a strong desire to help others, good listening skills, strong ethics, and the ability to work independently or as part of a team.

EXPLORING

There are many ways to learn more about a career as a rehabilitation counselor. You can visit the websites of college rehabilitation counseling programs to learn about typical classes and possible career paths, read books and journals about the field, and ask your teacher or school counselor to arrange an information interview with a rehabilitation counselor. Professional associations can also provide information about the field. Contact the associations listed at the end of this article for more information on education and careers.

EMPLOYERS

Approximately 129,500 rehabilitation counselors are employed in the United States. State and federal rehabilitation agencies, as well as community rehabilitation agencies, are major employers of counselors. Other employers include universities and other academic settings, substance abuse rehabilitation centers, correctional facilities, halfway houses, insurance companies, and independent-living centers.

There are many opportunities for rehabilitation counselors in related careers such as job placement specialist, general counselor, rehabilitation consultant, independent living specialist, and case manager.

GETTING A JOB

Many rehabilitation counselors obtain their first jobs as a result of contacts made through networking events, college internships, and career fairs. Others seek assistance in obtaining job leads from college career services offices, employment websites, and newspaper want ads. Additionally, the National Clearinghouse of Rehabilitation Training Materials provides job listings at its website, RehabJobs.org. Those interested in positions with the federal government should visit the U.S. Office of Personnel Management's website, www.usajobs.opm.gov.

ADVANCEMENT

Rehabilitation counselors advance by receiving salary increases and taking on managerial duties. Some counselors choose to work for their state's department of human services or work as supervisors or administrators. Others go into private practice or become college professors.

EARNINGS

Salaries for rehabilitation counselors vary by type of employer, geographic region, and the worker's experience, education, and skill level. Median annual salaries for rehabilitation counselors were $31,210 in 2009, according to the U.S. Department of Labor (USDL). Salaries ranged from less than $20,440 to $55,580 or more. The USDL reports the following mean annual earnings for rehabilitation counselors by employer: general medical and surgical hospitals, $47,740; state government, $44,190; local government, $39,590; vocational rehabilitation services, $31,820; individual and family services, $31,490; and residential mental retardation, mental health and substance abuse facilities, $29,220.

Rehabilitation counselors usually receive benefits such as health and life insurance, vacation days, sick leave, and a savings and pension plan. Self-employed workers must provide their own benefits.

EMPLOYMENT OUTLOOK

Employment for rehabilitation counselors is expected to grow faster than the average for all careers through 2018, according to the U.S. Department of Labor. The increasing number of elderly people (who typically become disabled or injured at a higher average rate than people in other demographic groups) will create good employment prospects for rehabilitation counselors. Growth will also occur as more elderly people are treated for mental health-related disabilities.

FOR MORE INFORMATION

For information on certification and the job search, contact
American Counseling Association
5999 Stevenson Avenue
Alexandria, VA 22304-3304
800-347-6647
www.counseling.org

For information about rehabilitation counseling, contact
American Rehabilitation and Counseling Association
www.arcaweb.org

For information on certification, contact
Commission on Rehabilitation Counselor Certification
1699 East Woodfield Road, Suite 300
Schaumburg, IL 60173-4957

847-944-1325
info@crccertification.com
www.crccertification.com

For information on accredited programs, contact
Council for Accreditation of Counseling and Related Educational Programs
American Counseling Association
1001 North Fairfax Street, Suite 510
Alexandria, VA 22314-1587
703-535-5990
www.cacrep.org

For information on approved programs, contact
Council on Rehabilitation Education
1699 East Woodfield Road, Suite 300
Schaumburg, IL 60173-4957
847-944-1345
www.core-rehab.org

continued on page 206

continued from page 205

For certification information, contact
National Board for
Certified Counselors
3 Terrace Way, Suite D
Greensboro, NC 27403-3660
www.nbcc.org

For information on rehabilitation
counseling, contact the following
organizations
National Clearinghouse of
Rehabilitation Training Materials
Utah State University
6524 Old Main Hill
Logan, UT 84322-6524
http://ncrtm.org

National Rehabilitation Association
633 South Washington Street
Alexandria, VA 22314-4109
703-836-0850
info@nationalrehab.org
www.nationalrehab.org

National Rehabilitation
Counseling Association
PO Box 4480
Manassas, VA 20108-4480
703-361-2077
info@nrca-net.org
http://nrca-net.org

Interview: Jeanne B. Patterson

Jeanne B. Patterson, Ed.D., CRC is a rehabilitation counselor who
resides in Tallahassee, Florida, and works in both North Florida and
South Georgia. She also serves as the administrator for the National
Rehabilitation Counseling Association. Jeanne discussed her career and
the field of rehabilitation counseling with the editors of *Hot Health Care*
Careers.

Q. Where do you work? How long have you worked in the field?

A.   For almost 35 years I have worked in different capacities as a rehabilitation counselor. Currently I am a self-employed rehabilitation counselor
and work as a sub-contractor for companies providing rehabilitation
counseling services to veterans who receive services from the Department
of Veterans Affairs (DVA). I am also a contractor for the Division of Blind
Services and Division of Vocational Rehabilitation, where I conduct vocational assessments of individuals with disabilities. The type of service
(e.g., assessment, placement, case management) I provide to veterans
varies with the referrals that I receive from rehabilitation counselors who
are employed by the DVA. Some veterans need assistance with getting a
job, whereas other veterans need assistance in exploring various career
options. For those veterans who are unable to work, I may be asked to
conduct an independent-living assessment to identify the services and/or
technology that are needed by the veterans.

Q. What made you want to enter this career?

A.   With an undergraduate major in psychology, I always knew I wanted to
work with people. When I learned about and enrolled in a graduate pro-

gram in rehabilitation counseling, I knew that I had found a wonderful fit. The course work, as well as practicum and internship, provided me with opportunities to make sure I was on the right career path. Over the years, there was never any doubt that helping individuals with disabilities to achieve independence, employment, and full integration into communities was an extremely rewarding career and the right career for me.

Q.   What is one thing that young people may not know about a career in rehabilitation counseling?

A.   One of the best parts of a career in rehabilitation counseling is the opportunity to work in diverse settings with individuals with various types of disabilities. If one chooses to do so, one can specialize by (1) the type of service provided (e.g., assessment, job development and placement, case management); (2) the type of disability (e.g., spinal cord injury, traumatic brain injury, autism, intellectual disability, emotional disability); and (3) the setting in which services are provided (e.g., state vocational rehabilitation agency, rehabilitation hospital, Department of Veterans Affairs, community-based rehabilitation programs, schools, workers' compensation). Also, one can change these areas throughout one's career. At this stage in my career, I have elected to be self-employed because of the flexibility it provides me, and I like working with individuals with diverse or multiple disabilities.

Q.   What are the most important personal and professional qualities for people in your career?

A.   First and foremost, one must like working with and have respect for all people. One must be non-judgmental and have empathy for people from all areas of life. All rehabilitation counselors are committed to helping people with disabilities achieve their goals. A critical part of being a counselor is having good listening and observational skills, which are part of counseling skills. A rehabilitation counselor must be committed to lifelong learning; the field of rehabilitation counseling is constantly evolving with new medical treatments and new services. One must have high ethical standards and use his or her knowledge and skills to help others.

Q.   What are some of the pros and cons of your job?

A.   The pros of the job include the ability to work in a range of settings with a diverse group of individuals with very different types of disabilities, whose ages cross the lifespan. One can move from one community or state to another and always find rehabilitation positions. Also, there are a variety of career ladders in most organizations and agencies that employ rehabilitation counselors.

The major con is that salaries in the human-service professions, including rehabilitation counseling, tend to be low. If making a large salary is a goal, then rehabilitation counseling may not be a good fit.

Q.   What advice would you give to young people who are interested in becoming rehabilitation counselors?

A.   Any person who is interested in becoming a rehabilitation counselor is encouraged to do some volunteer work with individuals with disabilities and ideally to volunteer with more than one agency or organization. Job

Other Fast-Growing Health Care Careers

The U.S. Department of Labor reports that the following careers will also enjoy strong employment growth from 2008 to 2018:

✔ Occupational Therapist Assistants and Aides: +30 percent

✔ Medical Equipment Repairers: +27 percent

✔ Pharmacy Technicians and Aides: +25 percent

✔ Optometrists: +24 percent

✔ Respiratory Therapists: +21 percent

✔ Chiropractors: +20 percent

✔ Massage Therapists: +19 percent

✔ Health Educators: +18 percent

✔ Recreational Therapists: +15 percent

✔ Clinical Laboratory Technologists and Technicians: +14 percent

shadowing rehabilitation counselors in a variety of settings offers insight into both the roles and the activities of rehabilitation counselors. Individuals who are interested in becoming rehabilitation counselors should not worry about specialization too early in their career exploration. One can major in a variety of undergraduate degrees prior to seeking admission to a master's degree program in rehabilitation counseling (e.g., psychology, social work, human services, special education). Also, there are a number of undergraduate programs in rehabilitation services or disability studies that provide early exposure to working with people with disabilities, and these provide an internship so that students have an opportunity to practice the knowledge and skills they have learned. A master's degree is required to be a rehabilitation counselor.

Q.   What is the employment outlook for rehabilitation counselors? How is the field changing?

A.   The employment outlook for rehabilitation counselors is excellent. According to the *Occupational Outlook Handbook,* the projected growth of jobs for rehabilitation counselors ranges from 14 to 19 percent from 2008-2018. Because there are not enough rehabilitation counselors for all the jobs available, some undergraduate programs in rehabilitation services/disability studies, as well as graduate programs in rehabilitation counseling, have grants to increase the number of individuals available to work in the state-federal vocational rehabilitation program. These grants usually help defray the cost of tuition for students and provide an incentive for individuals to pursue careers in rehabilitation counseling.

SPEECH-LANGUAGE PATHOLOGISTS AND AUDIOLOGISTS

OVERVIEW

Speech-language pathologists, also known as *speech therapists,* assess, diagnose, and treat people with voice disorders including speech, language, cognitive-communication, and fluency irregularities. *Audiologists* work with people who have hearing, balance, and other related ear problems. Speech-language pathologists need a master's degree in speech-language pathology to work in the field. Audiologists must have a doctorate in audiology to become certified. Approximately 119,300 speech-language pathologists and 12,800 audiologists are employed in the United States. Employment for speech therapists and audiologists is expected to be favorable through 2018.

THE JOB

People who suffer from illnesses and injuries involving hearing loss, and those with speech rhythm and fluency problems, developmental delays, or physical delays or disorders, often seek out the services of speech-language pathologists. These include patients with brain injury or deterioration, developmental delays or disorders, stroke, learning disabilities, cleft palate, voice pathology,

---

FAST FACTS

High School Subjects
Biology
Health
Speech

Personal Skills
Communication
Complex problem solving
Helping
Technical

Minimum Education Level
Master's degree
(speech-language pathologists)
Doctorate (audiologists)

Salary Range
$42,000 to $65,000 to
$101,000+ (speech-language
pathologists)
$40,000 to $63,000 to
$100,000+ (audiologists)

Employment Outlook
Faster than the average
(speech-language pathologists)
Much faster than the average
(audiologists)

O*NET-SOC
29-1127.00 (speech-language
pathologists)
29-1121.00 (audiologists)

GOE
14.06.01

DOT
076

NOC
3141

cerebral palsy, mental retardation, and emotional problems. These problems can be acquired, developmental, or congenital. Speech-language pathologists assess, diagnose, treat, and in some cases, prevent further damage or delays.

When working with a new patient, speech-language pathologists use written and oral tests to assess the nature and extent of the impairment. They also use special technology such as electronic speech fluency rating instruments for patients with fluency irregularities such as stammering or stuttering.

After diagnosis, speech-language pathologists create an individualized plan of care. They start patients on a regular therapy treatment schedule, the length and scope depending on the patient and his or her condition. Some treatments include breathing exercises or oral motor exercises to strengthen muscles that are used in swallowing and speaking. Speech therapists also teach patients how to form their mouth and tongue, by demonstration, in order to achieve different sounds. Patients with hearing loss or cochlear implants can be trained to use special audio devices for the telephone. Others may be taught to use sign language or other alternative communication methods. Treatments are also tailored to the patient's age. For example, when working with young children with cognitive communication disorders or speech delays, speech-language pathologists may incorporate games with repetitive exercises specially designed to hold a child's interest and attention span.

Many speech-language pathologists also work with patients who want to correct their speech rhythm and fluency problems. Some patients who depend on their voices for a living may seek help to erase an accent or reduce harshness in their voices. Others, such as transgender patients, often use speech therapy to change the pitch of their voices. Some speech-language pathologists are employed by businesses to help employees improve communication with their customers.

Speech-language pathologists in medical settings often consult with doctors, nurses, psychologists, and other therapists and health care workers when evaluating a new patient. In schools, they work closely with teachers, social workers, interpreters, and other professionals. Speech therapists stay in close contact with them throughout the course of therapy, as well as with patients and their families. Speech-language pathologists keep detailed records of patients' diagnosis, treatments and therapies, and continuing progress.

Audiologists work with people who have hearing loss, balance problems, or other issues concerning the ear. These conditions can be the result of injury, illness, infections, birth defects, exposure to loud noises, or simply advanced age.

When working with a new patient, audiologists use a battery of hearing tests to determine the level of impairment. They often consult with doctors, nurses, teachers, and family members to get a clearer picture of the patient's situation. Treatments include a thorough cleaning of the ear canal, as sometime excess wax may hinder hearing. Audiologists may suggest hearing devices or cochlear implants to improve a patient's hearing level. Audiologists also help patients adjust for hearing impairment by training them in the use of various hearing instruments or providing them with strategies to improve their listening skills. Some patients may be trained in lip reading. Audiologists may also encourage patients to use large area amplification devices or alerting devices in their homes.

Some people suffer from hearing loss due to their work environment. Patients include musicians and factory workers with work-related hearing problems. Audiologists try to prevent such injuries by measuring noise levels at the workplace. With extreme situations, they may suggest that clients wear protective ear devices to reduce excessive noise.

Speech-language pathologists and audiologists also are responsible for completing paperwork, billing, and supervising assistants and other staff. In addition to their clinical work, some speech-language pathologists and audiologists teach at the university level or conduct research on a particular specialty.

Full-time speech-language pathologists and audiologists work 40 hours a week, though most work longer hours in order to accommodate high patient loads. Some evening and weekend hours should be expected. Speech-language pathologists and audiologists who work part-time at several facilities need a reliable vehicle in order to travel from site to site.

Speech-language pathologists and audiologists who work in private practice have the added expense of overhead costs, including office space, furniture and equipment, and staff salary and benefits.

Speech-language pathologists and audiologists work in a wide range of settings, including schools, hospital rooms, rehabilitation centers, clinics, doctor's offices, and private practice (in office settings and in a patient's home). Their offices are located indoors and are clean and comfortable. A quiet atmosphere is often needed when working with patients. Speech-language pathologists and audiologists must relate to patients and their families, often explaining complicated medical terminology or treatments, or updating them on the patient's development and progress. They also consult with other health care professionals regarding patients.

REQUIREMENTS

HIGH SCHOOL

In high school, take courses in biology, anatomy and physiology, physics, mathematics, the social sciences, speech, English, languages, and psychology.

POSTSECONDARY TRAINING

The minimum educational requirement to work as a speech therapist is a master's degree in speech-language pathology. The Council on Academic Accreditation (CAA) has accredited approximately 265 graduate-level academic programs in speech-language pathology.

Audiologists need a doctorate in audiology (known as the Au.D.) to become certified. The CAA also accredits education programs in audiology. Approximately 75 doctoral programs in audiology are accredited by the organization. Typical classes for audiologists include Acquisition and Development of Speech and Language, Electrophysiology, Audiological Assessment and Diagnosis. Acoustic Phonetics, Auditory Disorders, Application of Hearing Aids to Auditory Disorders, Sign Language, and Ethical Issues in Audiology.

Both speech therapists and audiologists participate in clinical rotations during their college study. These become progressively more challenging and involve less direct supervision as the student proceeds in the program.

The American Speech-Language-Hearing Association offers a list of schools that award degrees in speech pathology and audiology at its website, www.asha.org/students/academic/EdFind.

Did You Know?

✔ Hearing loss affects one in 10 people in the United States—or about 31 million people.

✔ Ninety-five percent of people with hearing loss can be helped with hearing aids.

✔ Some of the risk factors for hearing loss include childhood infectious diseases (such as measles and mumps), recurrent ear infections, exposure to extremely loud noises, use of certain medications, and concussion and skull fracture.

Source: Audiology Foundation of America

CERTIFICATION AND LICENSING

Certification for speech-language pathologists and audiologists is available from the American Speech-Language-Hearing Association. Applicants must meet educational requirements, complete a supervised clinical practicum, and pass an examination, among other requirements. Speech therapists who complete these requirements are awarded the certificate of clinical competence in speech-language pathology, while audiologists receive the certificate of clinical competence in audiology. In addition, board certification in audiology is offered by the American Board of Audiology (www.americanboardofaudiology.org). The Board also offers specialty certification in cochlear implants. Those who obtain professional credentialing may satisfy some or all state licensing requirements. Speech-language pathologists with advanced training can become board recognized in child language, fluency disorders, and swallowing and swallowing disorders. Visit www.asha.org/students for more information.

Nearly all states regulate speech-language pathologists. According to the U.S. Department of Labor, "typical licensing requirements are a master's degree from an accredited college or university; a passing score on the national examination on speech-language pathology, offered through the Praxis Series of the Educational Testing Service; 300 to 375 hours of supervised clinical experience; and nine months of postgraduate professional clinical experience." Contact your state's regulatory board for information on regulation and eligibility requirements. Speech-language pathologists who work in public schools may need to meet additional licensing requirements. Check with your state's department of education for more information.

All states require audiologists to be licensed. Nearly 20 states require applicants to have a doctoral degree in audiology as a condition of licensure. Some states may also require audiologists to acquire a separate hearing-aid dispenser license. Contact your state's medical or health board for information on licensing requirements in your state.

OTHER REQUIREMENTS

Since they work with patients of all ages, speech-language pathologists and audiologists must be able to work with people who have a variety of personalities and attention spans. Successful professionals are able to stay patient and focused, with great attention to detail. They need excellent communication skills in order to write reports, interact with coworkers, and discuss test results and treatment plans with patients and their families. Other important traits include strong organizational skills, scientific aptitude, an empathetic personality, good listening skills, and a willingness to continue to learn about new diagnostic and treatment technologies throughout one's career.

Approximately 40 percent of speech-language pathologists and 15 percent of audiologists are members of a union or covered by a union contract.

EXPLORING

There are many ways to learn more about a career as a speech therapist or audiologist. You can read books and journals about the field, ask your teacher or school counselor to arrange an information interview with a speech therapist or audiologist, and visit the websites of college speech-language pathology or audiology programs to learn about typical classes and possible career paths. Professional associations can also provide information about the field. The American Speech-Language-Hearing Association provides a wealth of information on education and careers, as well as profiles of workers, at its website, www.asha.org/students. You should also try to land a part-time job in a setting that employs speech-language pathologists or audiologists. This will give you a chance to interact with these professionals and see if the career is a good fit for your interests and abilities.

EMPLOYERS

Approximately 119,300 speech-language pathologists are employed in the United States. Nearly 50 percent work in educational services. Others are employed by health maintenance organizations; hospitals; public health departments; research agencies; nursing care facilities; home health care services; individual and family services; outpatient care centers; child day care centers; long-term care facilities; rehabilitation centers; government agencies; and corporate speech-language pathology programs. About nine percent of speech therapists are self-employed.

About 12,800 audiologists are employed in the United States. Approximately 64 percent work in health care facilities. These include offices of physicians or other health practitioners, outpatient care centers, and hospitals. About 14 percent work in educational services. Other employment settings include health and personal care stores and government agencies. Some audiologists work as audiology professors, as designers of hearing instruments and testing equipment, and in industrial settings (such as factories) creating hearing conservation programs for workers.

GETTING A JOB

Many speech-language pathologists and audiologists obtain their first jobs as a result of contacts made through college internships, career fairs, or networking events. Others seek assistance in obtaining job leads from college career services offices, newspaper want ads, and employment websites. Additionally, the American Speech-Language-Hearing Association provides job listings and career advice (such as preparing a résumé, acing a job interview, and negotiating a salary) at its website, www.asha.org/careers/job. Those interested in positions with the federal government should visit the U.S. Office of Personnel Management's website, www.usajobs.opm.gov.

ADVANCEMENT

Speech-language pathologists and audiologists advance by receiving pay raises, by taking on managerial or administrative duties, by becoming college professors, and by becoming experts in certain populations (such as youth or the elderly) or disorders (such as learning disabilities). Others open their own practices.

EARNINGS

Salaries for speech-language pathologists and audiologists vary by type of employer, geographic region, and the worker's experience, education, and skill level. Median annual salaries for speech-language pathologists were $65,090 in 2009, according to the U.S. Department of Labor (USDL). Salaries ranged from less than $42,310 to $101,820 or more. The USDL reports the following mean annual earnings for speech-language pathologists by employer: home health care services, $87,820; nursing care facilities, $80,500; community care facilities for the elderly, $79,130; offices of other health practitioners, $74,810; general medical and surgical hospitals, $72,030; and elementary and secondary schools, $62,860.

Speech-language pathologists who worked in health care earned average salaries of $70,000 in 2009, according to the American Speech-Language-Hearing Association. Those employed in administration earned from less than $72,800 to $100,000 or more.

Audiologists earned salaries that ranged from less than $40,650 to $100,480 in 2009, according to the USDL. They earned a median annual salary of $63,230.

Employers offer a variety of benefits, including the following: medical, dental, and life insurance; paid holidays, vacations, and sick and personal days; 401(k) plans; profit-sharing plans; retirement and pension plans; and educational-assistance programs. Self-employed and part-time workers must provide their own benefits. Approximately 20 percent of speech-language pathologists work part-time.

EMPLOYMENT OUTLOOK

Employment for speech-language pathologists is expected to grow by 19 percent from 2008 to 2018, according to the U.S. Department of Labor (USDL)—or faster than the average for all careers. Increases in elementary- and secondary-school enrollments, the aging of the large Baby Boomer generation (which will have a growing number of neurological disorders and associated language, speech, and swallowing impairments), and medical advances that are increasing survival rates for trauma and stroke victims and premature infants (who may require speech therapy) are all increasing demand for speech-language pathologists. Demand will be best for speech-language pathologists who speak a second language, such as Spanish, and who are willing to relocate to areas of the United States where demand is higher for speech therapists.

Job opportunities for audiologists are expected to grow much faster than the average for all occupations through 2018, according to the USDL. But since only a small number of people are employed in the field, it will be difficult to land a job. Those who have the Au.D. degree will have the best job prospects. As school enrollments continue to grow, there will be good job prospects for audiologists who work at elementary and secondary schools. Areas that have a large number of retirees, who typically have more hearing problems than other demographic groups, will also offer strong prospects for audiologists.

FOR MORE INFORMATION

For information on hearing and balance disorders, contact
American Auditory Society
19 Mantua Road
Mt. Royal, NJ 08061-1006
www.amauditorysoc.org

For a wealth of information on education and careers in speech-language pathology and audiology, visit the association's website.

American Speech-Language-Hearing Association
2200 Research Boulevard
Rockville, MD 20850-3289
actioncenter@asha.org
www.asha.org

For information on the Au.D. degree, contact
Audiology Foundation of America
8 North 3rd Street, Suite 301
Lafayette, IN 47901-1276
www.audfound.org

continued on page 216

continued from page 215

For information on audiologists who work in education and other settings, contact

Educational Audiology Association
3030 West 81st Avenue
Westminster, CO 80031-4111
admin@edaud.org
www.edaud.org

This association is for undergraduate and graduate students studying normal and disordered human communication. Visit its website for more information.

National Student Speech Language Hearing Association
2200 Research Boulevard, #450
Rockville, MD 20850-3289
nsslha@asha.org
www.nsslha.org

Interview: Diane Paul

Dr. Diane Paul is the director of clinical issues in speech-language pathology at the American Speech-Language-Hearing Association. She discussed her career and the field with the editors of *Hot Health Care Careers*.

Q.   What made you want to enter this career?

A.   I heard a camp counselor talking about the field of speech-language pathology. When I needed to select a major, I was going through the course catalogue and came across some speech-language pathology courses. Although my entry into the field may have been based more on a need to find a major rather than a life calling, my interest and desire to stay in the field has been sustained because of my passion for the varied, interesting, and rewarding work.

Q.   What is one thing that young people may not know about a career as a speech-language pathologist?

A.   The settings (school, hospital, university, private-practice clinic), clients (children and adults across the life span), types of communication disorders (speech-articulation, voice, fluency; language-understanding and expression in the areas of vocabulary, grammar, use of words in social situations, reading, and writing; and swallowing disorders), and nature of work (clinic, research, teaching, administration) are so varied, that the work can easily maintain a person's interest for a lifetime.

Q.   What are the most important personal and professional qualities for people in your career?

A.   Energy, enthusiasm, skills in spoken and written communication, enjoyment interacting with different people, sensitivity to the needs of persons with communication disorders, and organization

Q. What do you like most and least about your job?

A. Most: Each day is different and I have the opportunity to do creative, intellectually stimulating, meaningful work that makes a difference. Least: Not enough time in the day to accomplish all that I'd like to do.

Q. What advice would you give to young people who are interested in the field?

A. The population in our country is increasingly diverse. Knowing at least one other language besides English would be helpful to serve a broader population. Developing cultural competence is necessary to serve a broad population as well.

Q. What is the employment outlook for your field? How will the field change in the future?

A. We are serving individuals across the age span with more severe medical needs. For example, more infants are surviving with lower birth weights and resulting complications, including language and learning problems. People are living longer and may have communication needs resulting from strokes, injuries, or other health conditions.

We also are serving individuals without communication disorders who want to improve the effectiveness of their communication in the workplace or other settings.

Technological advances are changing the way we provide services: there are opportunities for telepractice; individuals with more severe disabilities are benefiting from the new computers and other speech-generating devices as an augmentative or alternative form of communication.

Services are becoming more collaborative: speech-language pathologists work on teams with parents, teachers, and other professionals. They collaborate on the development and implementation of the individualized education program.

Our scope of practice has expanded over the years and likely will continue to change. We've moved from a field focused primarily on speech correction to one with a much greater focus on language, communication, swallowing, literacy, social interactions, learning and learning disabilities, severe disabilities, and other specialized areas.

Currently, we are experiencing shortages of speech-language pathologists in the United States. The Bureau of Labor Statistics indicates that speech-language pathology is one of the best professions for seeking a job.

Interview: Pamela Mason

Pamela Mason, M.Ed., CCC-A is the director of audiology professional practices at the American Speech-Language-Hearing Association. She discussed her career and the field of audiology with the editors of *Hot Health Care Careers*.

Q. What made you want to enter this career?

A. I learned about the profession of audiology when I enrolled in an undergraduate program in speech-language pathology. It was then that I realized that I might have what it takes to become a good audiologist. I have always enjoyed music and was never afraid of audio technology; back then I felt confident setting up a stereo and understood (somehow through my music interest) how to set the frequency equalizer and volume for best fidelity.

I also have good communication skills and love to teach. Both of these qualities are necessary to become a good audiologist and to enjoy the profession. Audiologists must be able to communicate with and teach individuals (patients and clients) with hearing or balance issues. It takes empathy as well. An audiologist understands the impact of hearing loss on the quality of life. The audiologist must have good listening skills, which are part of counseling. If you are working with infants and young children, and hearing loss has been identified at birth during universal newborn hearing screening programs in hospitals, these skills are paramount because it can be difficult news to accept when your baby is only one day old. Young families need support and information. Audiologists also need to be objective in interpreting test results and in their support of patients/clients. Decisions are never based just upon the audiologist's thoughts; options are discussed, and the families with knowledge makes the decision.

Q.   What is the one thing that young people may not know about a career in audiology?

A.   Wow! What a question! Our services are necessary across a lifetime. More than 95 percent of infants born in the United States receive a hearing screening before they are discharged from the hospital. Infants identified [with hearing loss] through the screening are followed through a process called Early Hearing Detection and Intervention (EHDI). Pediatric audiologists work with families, infants, pediatricians, and other health professionals in the EHDI programs in each state. On the other end of the age continuum, the baby boomers are approaching retirement, and hearing loss in the older population is greater than in younger individuals. And over the past decade or so, the scope of practice has grown and will continue to grow. Audiologists are also expert in understanding the balance system, which is situated in the inner ear next to the cochlea, the end organ for hearing. Audiologists help people with balance concerns. Through a battery of tests, audiologists can assist in the medical diagnosis of the cause of balance disorders.

Employment opportunities are expected to grow. A four-year postbaccalaureate degree is required. Detailed career information is available at www.asha.org; look in the student tab on the left column.

Q.   What are the most important personal and professional qualities for people in your career?

A.

✔ Work with people of all ages
✔ Enjoy technology
✔ Work in a variety of settings
✔ Assess, diagnosis, and treat individuals with non-medical hearing and balance problems
✔ Good communication skills

✔ Good listening skills

✔ Objective when faced with difficult situations

Q. What do you like most about your job?

A. Every day is different! Each patient brings a new set of unique character-istics—both as an individual and as an individual with a hearing or bal-ance concern. I like helping people. Audiology is not a life-saving profes-sion, but it is a life-changing profession.

Q. What advice would you give to young people who are interested in the field?

A. In a word: Google. And begin your Internet search at www.asha.org. Through our website, you can locate an audiologist nearby your home at www.asha.org/proserv. Contact that person, and learn firsthand about the field.

Q. How will the field change in the future?

A. Audiology is a dynamic field with new technological advances occurring frequently. The following areas may be considered new areas of clinical practice based on a review of data sources.

✔ New treatment protocols for tinnitus treatment

✔ Caloric stimulation for balance treatment

✔ Genetic screening for hearing loss

✔ Hybrid cochlear implants

✔ Preservation of hearing using otoprotective agents

SURGICAL TECHNOLOGISTS

OVERVIEW

Surgical technologists help surgeons, nurses, and other members of the surgical team before, during, and after surgical procedures. They are sometimes referred to as *surgical technicians* or *operating room technicians*. Their duties include assisting surgeons and nurses during an operation and preparing the operating room and supplies before and after the procedure. Training programs for surgical technologists last nine to 24 months and lead to a certificate, diploma, or associate's degree. Approximately 91,500 surgical technologists are employed in the United States. Employment for surgical technologists is expected to grow much faster than the average for all careers through 2018.

THE JOB

You've probably seen enough

FAST FACTS

High School Subjects
Biology
Health

Personal Skills
Communication
Coordination
Critical thinking
Operation monitoring

Minimum Education Level
Some postsecondary training

Salary Range
$27,000 to $39,000 to $55,000+

Employment Outlook
Much faster than the average

O*NET-SOC
29-2055.00

GOE
14.05.01

DOT
079

NOC
3219

operating-room scenes on television and in the movies to know that there are many health care professionals present during a surgery—far more than just surgeons and nurses. Surgical technologists are part of this group. Preparing the operating room, creating and maintaining the sterile field, and gathering and organizing necessary equipment and supplies are just some of the vital pre-operative responsibilities of this professional. During surgery, the surgical technologist passes instruments to the surgeon and must be skilled enough to anticipate the needs of the surgeon. He or she also handles and prepares medications and specimens. When the surgery has concluded, the surgical technologist is responsible for maintaining the sterile field until the patient is transported and removing any instruments or equipment. The operating room can be a stressful environment, and the surgical technologist must be able to work well under pressure. The surgical technologist's role is indeed vital to a successful surgery—he or she plays a role in saving lives. The following paragraphs provide an overview of the most popular surgical technology specialties.

Scrub surgical technologists assist the surgical team during procedures. They have a good understanding of the type and scope of the procedure being done and are able to foresee the needs of the medical team. For pre-operative case management, their duties include preparing the operating room. This entails making sure all supplies are readily available and equipment is functioning properly. Scrub surgical technologists wear operating gowns and gloves only after they have scrubbed—washing thoroughly with antiseptic soap. They set up the sterile table and make sure supplies, instruments, medications, and solutions are in place. They keep an accurate count of all pieces of equipment and supplies, such as forceps, sponges, or rolls of gauze. The pre-operative count must match at the end of the procedure, ensuring no foreign objects are mistakenly left in the patient's body during surgery. This count is done with another member of the surgical team.

Scrub surgical technologists help doctors and nurses into their sterile gowns and gloves. They are also responsible for exposing the sterile area by draping the patient with cloth.

During the surgical procedure, scrub surgical technologists pass instruments to the surgeon. When the surgeon asks for a particular instrument, the technologist must be able to locate and give the instrument quickly, many times anticipating the needs of the surgeon. Technologists may also prepare sterile dressing in preparation for closing the surgical site. At this time, the post-operative count of instruments and dressings is made.

After the surgical procedure, scrub surgical technologists are responsible for terminal sterilization of all instruments and equipment used. This is important to ensure the instruments and equipments are free from all traces of bacteria. The technologist also cleans the operating room and prepares it for the next procedure.

Circulating surgical technologists have many of the same pre-operative and post-operative duties as scrub surgical technologists. They obtain necessary instruments, supplies, and equipment, and they help sterilize the operating room after each procedure. However, circulating surgical technologists have more patient responsibility. Before each procedure, they check the patient's chart and consent forms to match the proper patient with the surgical procedure that is scheduled. They then transport the patient to the operating room and transfer him or her to the operating table. Circulating surgical technologists often converse with the patient, and if he or she is anxious or fearful, they may provide words of reassurance and comfort.

Circulating surgical technologists apply electrosurgical grounding pads, monitors, or other equipment before the procedure begins. They also prepare the patient's skin with an antiseptic solution to ensure that bacteria does not enter the patient's body through the incision. When surgeons remove a piece of tissue for further pathology, circulating surgical technologists place the specimen in the proper solution and container. They also secure the patient's dressings while the surgeon closes the incision. Afterwards, circulating surgical technologists transfer the patient to the operating recovery room.

With advanced training and certification, surgical technologists can advance to the rank of *first assistant surgical technologist.* First assistant technologists help surgeons during procedures by carrying out many of the technical tasks. They hold instruments such as retractors or forceps, as instructed by the surgeon. They may also help in hemostasis—the process of stopping a bleed—by applying electrocautery or clamps. Some first assistant technologists may be directed by surgeons to cut suture material or apply dressings to a closed wound.

Second assistant surgical technologists handle technical tasks that do not involve cutting, clamping, and suturing tissue. They may hold retractors or instruments, use suction or sponges on the operative site, connect drains to suction apparatus, apply dressings to closed wounds, and perform other duties.

Full-time surgical technologists work 40 hours a week, with some shifts scheduled on weekends and holidays. Some surgical technologists have assigned emergency call shifts.

At times the work environment can be quite stressful, especially when assigned surgical procedures back-to-back. It is important for surgical technologists to stay alert and focused, paying special attention to key details. Surgical technologists are also exposed to many situations that may be unpleasant or uncomfortable, such as blood or open wounds. Exposure to communicable diseases is also possible.

REQUIREMENTS

HIGH SCHOOL

In high school, take courses in health, anatomy and physiology, biology, chemistry, and mathematics to prepare for the field. Speech classes will help you to develop your communication skills, which you will need when interacting with coworkers and patients.

POSTSECONDARY TRAINING

Training programs for surgical technologists last nine to 24 months and lead to a certificate, diploma, or associate's degree. Typical classes include Surgical Instrumentation, Equipment and Supplies, Principles of Asepsis and Sterile Technique, Surgical Procedures, Medical Terminology, Anatomy and Physiology, Microbiology, Surgical Pharmacology and Anesthesia Techniques, Safety Standards in the Operating Room, General Patient Care and Safety, Preoperative and Postoperative Considerations, and Legal, Moral, and Ethical Issues. Students also participate in clinical experiences under the supervision of trained surgical technologists. The Commission on Accreditation of Allied Health Education Programs (CAA-HEP) has accredited more than 450 surgical technology programs. Visit its website, www.caahep.org, for a list of programs.

CERTIFICATION AND LICENSING

Certification is available from the National Board of Surgical Technology and Surgical Assisting (www.nbstsa.org). Those who graduate from a CAA-

HEP-accredited program and pass a national certification examination can use the designation, certified surgical technologist. The certified surgical first assistant designation is also available. Surgical technologists can also become certified by the National Center for Competency Testing (www.ncctinc.com). Applicants who meet education and experience requirements and pass an examination may use the designation, tech in surgery-certified. Certification, while voluntary, is highly recommended. It is an excellent way to stand out from other job applicants and demonstrate your abilities to prospective employers.

OTHER REQUIREMENTS

To be a successful surgical technologist, you should be very organized and attentive to detail. You will need excellent manual dexterity, and you should be in good physical shape, since you will be on your feet for long periods of time and be required (in the case of circulating technologists) to move quickly back and forth between operating rooms and supply areas during surgeries. You must be able to respond quickly to requests for instruments; many experienced technologists are able to anticipate the instruments needed by a surgeon before they are even requested. Finally, you should be willing to continue to learn throughout your career via seminars, educational conferences, and other methods of continuing education.

EXPLORING

Does the career of surgical technologist sound interesting to you? If so, there are many ways to learn more about a career as a surgical technologist. You can read books and journals (such as *The Surgical Technologist,* www.ast.org/publications/journal.aspx) about the field, visit the websites of college surgical technology programs to learn about typical classes and possible career paths, and ask your teacher or school counselor to arrange an information interview with a surgical technologist. The Association of Surgical Technologists provides a wealth of information on education and careers at its website, www.ast.org.

EMPLOYERS

Approximately 91,500 surgical technologists are employed in the United States—with about 71 percent employed by hospitals, mainly in delivery and operating rooms. Other employers include outpatient care centers, offices of physicians and other medical professionals, and the U.S. military. Some surgical technologists work as college educators; others pursue careers in medical equipment sales.

GETTING A JOB

Many surgical technologists obtain their first jobs as a result of contacts made through college internships, career fairs, or networking events. Others seek assistance in obtaining job leads from college career services offices, newspaper want ads, and employment websites. Additionally, the

Association of Surgical Technologists provides job listings at its website, http://careercenter.ast.org/search.cfm. Those interested in positions with the federal government should visit the U.S. Office of Personnel Management's website, www.usajobs.opm.gov.

ADVANCEMENT

Surgical technologists advance by receiving salary increases and by specializing in a particular area of surgery, such as neurosurgery. Others become managers of surgical technologists or supervise central supply departments in hospitals. Surgical technologists who earn graduate degrees can become college professors. Many technologists complete additional education to become physician assistants.

EARNINGS

Salaries for surgical technologists vary by type of employer, geographic region, and the worker's experience, education, and skill level. Median annual salaries for surgical technologists were $39,400 in 2009, according to the U.S. Department of Labor (USDL). Salaries ranged from less than $27,910 to $55,620 or more. The USDL reports the following mean annual earnings for surgical technologists by employer: outpatient care centers, $41,320; offices of physicians, $41,260; general medical and surgical hospitals, $40,330; and offices of dentists, $38,060.

Surgical technologists usually receive benefits such as health and life insurance, vacation days, sick leave, and a savings and pension plan. Some employers offer tuition reimbursement and child care benefits. Part-time workers must provide their own benefits.

EMPLOYMENT OUTLOOK

According to the U.S. Department of Labor, the demand for surgical technologists is expected to increase by 25 percent through 2018, or much faster than the average for all occupations. An aging population along with advances in medical technology (such as fiber optics and laser technology) are creating demand for skilled surgical technologists. Hospitals, the largest employers of surgical technologists, will continue to offer a large number of job openings, but employment will grow fastest at offices of physicians and in outpatient care centers, including ambulatory surgical centers. Employment prospects will be best for surgical technologists who are certified and who are willing to relocate to areas of the country where there is a shortage of workers.

FOR MORE INFORMATION

For education and career information, contact
**Association of
Surgical Technologists**
6 West Dry Creek Circle, Suite 200
Littleton, CO 80120-8031
303-694-9130
www.ast.org

Interview: Kathleen Uribe

Kathleen Uribe is the program chair of the Surgical Technology Program at Southeast Community College in Lincoln, Nebraska. Students who complete the program receive an associate of applied science degree. Kathleen discussed the career of surgical technologist with the editors of *Hot Health Care Careers*.

Q. Can you tell us about the career of surgical technologist?

A. Surgical technologists are highly skilled and uniquely prepared to their role as a valuable and integral part of the surgical team. Surgical technologists perform a wide variety of tasks in the operating room. They anticipate the needs of the surgical team, handle instruments, and assist the surgeon by holding retractors, cutting sutures, suctioning wounds, adjusting lights, and applying dressings, to name a few. Additional responsibilities are to operate the sterilizer; set up the room in preparation for the procedure; care for and handle instruments before, during, and after the procedure; and to prepare for the next day's schedule. The primary focus is keeping patient care number one. The motto of the surgical technologist is, *Aeger Primo*—The Patient Comes First.

Q. What high school classes should students focus on to be successful in this major?

A. High school students should focus on the sciences, such as anatomy and physiology, biology, and microbiology.

Q. What are the most important personal and professional qualities for surgical technology students and professionals in the field?

A. A successful student and surgical technologist is highly motivated, is a self-starter, is honest, and has integrity. Technologists should be able to handle difficult and stressful situations. They also should be physically capable to stand for long periods of time and lift heavy objects.

Q. Where do surgical technology graduates find employment?

A. Job opportunities include hospitals, medical centers, surgery outpatient centers, doctor's offices, labor and delivery departments, the sterile processing and distribution department of a hospital, education departments, and medical sales, to name a few. Surgical technology is also a great stepping stone as preparation to become a physician's assistant. There is also the opportunity to advance to the position of first assistant. The certified first assistant's main responsibility is to assist the surgeon during surgery above and beyond the tasks and skills of the certified surgical technologist. Additional schooling and certification is required to function as a certified first assistant.

INDEX

ALSO FROM
COLLEGE & CAREER PRESS

BOOKS

Hot Jobs: More Than 25 Careers With the Highest Pay, Fastest Growth, and Most New Job Openings

Hot Jobs features more than 25 hot careers—careers that will pay the most, grow most quickly, and employ the largest number of people through 2018, according to the U.S. Department of Labor. Some of the hottest jobs include Computer Software Engineers, Civil Engineers, Computer Support Specialists, Computer Systems Analysts, Construction Managers, Market Research Analysts, Medical Scientists, Personal Financial Advisors, Pharmacists, Physical Therapists, Registered Nurses, and Kindergarten, Elementary, Middle School, and Special Education Teachers.

Each career article provides an overview of the job and typical work environments, educational requirements, personal skills, methods of exploring the career while still in high school, tips on landing a job, typical employers, information on the long-term employment outlook and hot specialties, and sources of additional information. The book also features nearly 40 interviews with professionals and educators, photographs, and useful sidebars that list books, websites, fun facts, and other helpful information.

ISBN-13: 978-0-9745251-6-7, 224 pages, $14.99, 7.25 x 9, Paperback or E-Book, Index

Nontraditional Careers for Women: More Than 25 Great Jobs for Women With Apprenticeships Through PhDs

Women are making great strides regarding gender equality and equal pay in the workplace. But there are many high-paying, fast-growing fields that young women still may not be aware of as exciting career options. The U.S. Department of Labor classifies nontraditional careers for women as those in which 25 percent or less of the people working in that particular career are female. Educational requirements for these rewarding jobs range from apprenticeship training to doctorate degrees. Nontraditional Careers for Women details 25 high-paying, fast-growing nontraditional career paths for women. Careers include Business Executive, Architect, Computer Software Engineer, Chiropractor, Police Officer, Industrial Engineer, Firefighter, Civil Engineer, Construction Manager, and Carpenter, Electrician, and Airplane Pilot.

In each career article, we provide an overview of the career and typical work environments, recommended high school classes and activities, educational requirements, personal skills, methods of exploring the career while still in high school, tips on landing a job, typical employers, information on the employment outlook and hot specialties, and contact information for professional associations. The book also features interviews with women who have excelled in these careers. They provide useful advice to young women contemplating careers in nontraditional fields. Other features include photographs and useful sidebars that feature books, websites, fun facts about the field, and other helpful information.

ISBN-13: 978-0-9745251-9-8, 192 pages, $17.99, Paperback or EBook, 6 x 9, Indexes

They Teach That in College series

Looking for information about out-of-the ordinary, cutting-edge college majors? Our **They Teach That in College!?** series will help you learn more about interesting and unique college majors and programs that will provide young people with great job prospects in the next decade. Each book in the **They Teach That in College!?** series provides information about lucrative and cutting-edge college majors unknown to many counselors, educators, and parents. Majors include Bioinformatics, Broadcast Meteorology, Comic Book Art, Entrepreneurship, Horticultural

Therapy, Mechatronics Systems Engineering, Motorsports Engineering, Music Therapy, Nanotechnology, Renewable Energy, Satellite Communications, Sustainable Agriculture, and Toy Design. Each title provides descriptions of these majors, contact information for colleges and universities that offer these majors, lists of typical classes and employers, interesting sidebars, and interviews with college professors.

They Teach That in College: A Resource Guide to More Than 95 Interesting College Majors, 2nd Edition

ISBN-10: 0-9745251-7-0, ISBN-13: 978-0-9745251-7-4, 352 pages, $14.99, PB, 6 x 9, Indexes, Photographs

They Teach That in Community College: A Resource Guide to 70 Interesting College Majors and Programs

ISBN-10: 0-9745251-2-X, ISBN-13: 978-0-9745251-2-9, 320 pages, $9.99, PB, 6 x 9, Indexes, Photographs

They Teach That in College-Midwest Edition: A Resource Guide to More Than 65 Interesting College Majors

ISBN-10: 0-9745251-3-8, ISBN-13: 978-0-9745251-3-6, 320 pages, $9.99, PB, 6 x 9, Indexes, Photographs. This book provides coverage of college programs (at 580 colleges) in Illinois, Indiana, Iowa, Kansas, Michigan, Minnesota, Missouri, Nebraska, North Dakota, Ohio, South Dakota, and Wisconsin.

NEWSLETTERS

CAM Report newsletter

The **CAM Report** is a career resource newsletter geared toward guidance and education professionals and the students they serve. Its mission: to provide time-saving, comprehensive resources to those who assist students with career discovery.

For Each Issue: ISSN: 0745-4341; published bimonthly September through May, and twice during the summer; 4 pages, 8.5 x 11, Two-Color

Subscription Rates: 1 year/$75 (20 issues); 2 years/$140 (40 issues); 3 years/$210 (60 issues)

College Spotlight newsletter

College Spotlight is a resource newsletter geared toward guidance and education professionals and the students they serve. Its mission: to help those concerned with selecting, applying to, evaluating, and entering college, as well as to provide other alternatives for today's high school graduates.

For Each Issue: ISSN 1525-4313, published six times during the school year, 12 pages, 8.5 x 11, Two-Color, Photographs

Subscription Rates: 1 year/$34.95 (9 issues); 2 years/$54.95 (18 issues); 3 years/$69.95 (27 issues)

Visit www.collegeandcareerpress.com to read introductions, tables of contents, and sample chapters or copies (newsletters) for all of our products.

5 Ways to Order:

Mail: College & Career Press, PO Box 300484, Chicago, IL 60630

Phone/Fax: 773/282-4671

amorkes@chicagopa.com

www.collegeandcareerpress.com